To Carton Bost Family
my best wishes
Marg devonis

PEOPLE OF FAITH
The Story of Hôtel-Dieu Grace Hospital
1888 to 2013

People of Faith

The Story of Hôtel-Dieu Grace Hospital
1888 to 2013

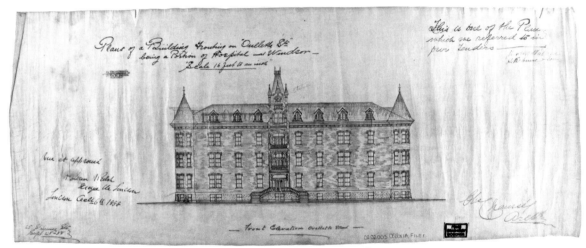

Marty Gervais

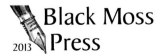

Black Moss Press 2013

© 2013 Marty Gervais

Library and Archives Canada Cataloguing in Publication

Gervais, Marty, 1946-, author
    People of faith : the story of Hôtel-Dieu Grace Hospital 1888-2013 / Marty Gervais.

Includes bibliographical references.
ISBN 978-0-88753-529-1 (bound)

    1. Hôtel-Dieu Grace Hospital (Windsor, Ont.). 2. Religious Hospitallers of St. Joseph.
3. Hospitals—Ontario—Windsor—History. I. Title.

RA983.W55H68 2013   362.1109713'32   C2013-905312-3

Cover: Architectural drawing of Hôtel-Dieu Hospital, 1888, Hôtel-Dieu Grace Hospital archives
Back Cover: Private hospital room, October 1918, Hôtel-Dieu Grace Hospital archives
Photos: Unless otherwise stated, photos are from Hôtel-Dieu Grace Hospital archives

Design: Karen Veryle Monck, Benchmark Publishing & Design Inc., Windsor, Ontario
Edited by: Brian Fox, Lisa Salfi, Jay Rankin, Jessica Knapp

Every effort has been made to secure permission for photographs and drawings reproduced in this book from the copyright holders. We regret any inadvertent omission.

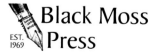 Black Moss
EST. 1969 Press

Published by Black Moss Press at 2450 Byng Road, Windsor, Ontario, N8W 3E8. Canada
Printed in Canada

Table of Contents

Introduction

COMPASSION, COMMITMENT, AND COURAGE CHARACTERIZE THIS BOOK ABOUT A GROUP OF WOMEN who founded Hotel-Dieu 125 years ago.

My involvement with the Religious Hospitallers of St. Joseph started in 1983 when I started working at Hôtel-Dieu Hospital in St. Catharines, Ontario. Then in 2002 I was appointed President and Chief Executive Officer of Hotel-Dieu Grace Hospital in Windsor. As all of you know life has interesting twists and turns and, in my case, I was asked by the Minister of Health and Long Term Care to return to Windsor in 2011 as the government appointed Supervisor of Hôtel-Dieu Grace Hospital. Effective January 5, 2011, I was appointed Supervisor through an Order-in-Council to act exclusively in the place of the board, its officers, and corporate members. Subsequent to this appointment the board asked me to stay on as President and Chief Executive Officer.

This book contextualizes and captures a remarkable 125-year journey by the Religious Hospitallers in Windsor, Ontario. In reading this, you are given a behind-the-scenes look at the women who established the hospital and the challenges that had to be overcome at that time and throughout the hospital's 125 years of service to this community. This account chronicles the people, the strategies, and the decisions that shaped the delivery of health care in Windsor and contributed to the evolution of a health care organization that adapted to changing circumstances and conditions.

Marty Gervais is ideally and uniquely qualified to write this book. His love of the city and his appreciation for the history of Windsor is unparalleled. For many years Marty wrote a must-read 'My Town' column in the Windsor Star that reflected his ability to and interest in capturing the ethos and the character of Windsor and the people who live here. In 2006 he wrote My Town: Faces of Windsor that captured the faces of this fine community. His ability to portray the key aspects of the history of the hospital and the Sisters is borne out in his 2005 book Taking My Blood that charted his time in a hospital.

If you are interested in Windsor, history, health care, or a story of compassion, commitment, and courage this is the book for you.

Ken Deane
President and Chief Executive Officer
of Hôtel-Dieu Grace Hospital

PART I

Beginnings

1888-1900

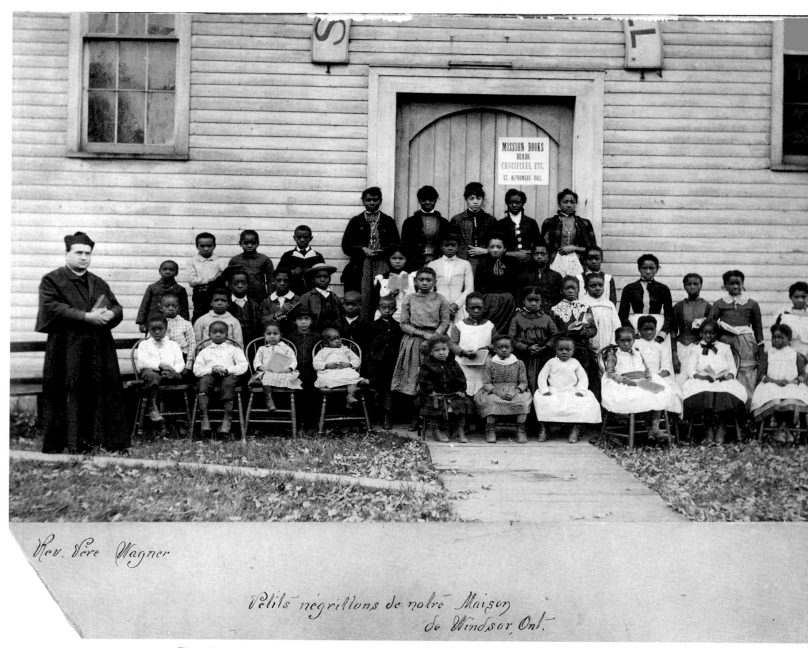

Rev. Père Wagner

Petits négrillons de notre Maison
de Windsor, Ont.

First class of the Mission for Coloured Children in 1888; Reverend J.T. Wagner stands on the left.

The Dream

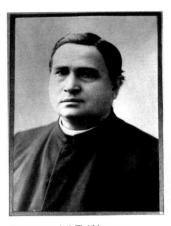

Reverend J.T. Wagner (1837-1896) Founder of St. Alphonsus Parish and Hôtel-Dieu Hospital, Windsor

THEY DIDN'T KNOW WHAT TO MAKE OF IT WHEN THEY STEPPED OFF THE TRAIN IN WINDSOR. THERE were five of them, all standing there looking a little bewildered that day, when a stout and beaming priest, Father James Theodore Wagner, greeted these religious sisters from Montreal on September 13, 1888. The train was several hours late. Father Wagner escorted the exhausted nuns in a horse-drawn carriage, and loaded it up with their heavy trunks and boxes laden with both medical and personal necessities. They headed to the Holy Names Sisters convent on Ouellette Avenue, where they rested before being feted to a hearty meal. The nuns spent their first night in Windsor at the convent.

The next morning, Father Wagner returned to escort the five sisters to St. Alphonsus Hall, the old barn-like former chapel on Goyeau Street. Another sister—Sister Odile—had arrived several days ahead to clean and prepare the place for their arrival. Father Wagner, the Catholic Church's dean of Essex and pastor of St. Alphonsus, had also repaired the roof. Apparently he also politely apologized for these quarters falling short of being the most ideal for them. He clearly did not calculate how long it would be before these sisters could have their own residence, a proper one connected to the proposed hospital.

The nuns admittedly were troubled. They had been dispatched to this frontier town by Mother Justine Bonneau, Superior of the Religious Hospitallers of St. Joseph, a cloistered community in Montreal. She had written to Father Wagner offering assistance after seeing a circular that had been mailed out to churches and communities all over the country in hopes of raising money to help the orphaned and unschooled children. In particular, Wagner wanted to find aid for the black population in his Windsor parish. So adamant and focused was he on this that he won the approval from Bishop John Walsh of the London Diocese to travel to Paris to speak to a crowd of 5,000. Bonneau reacted to the heart-felt appeal by sending him $2.50, but also informed the priest that if ever he envisioned building a hospital in Windsor, along with a proper school, her sisters—dedicated to caring for the sick and poor—could help. The idea immediately resonated with Wagner, because some civic leaders in Windsor had already voiced the necessity for a hospital. For one, Dr. Richard Carney, appointed as the city's physician (similar to a medical officer of health) tried to drum up interest in the establishment of a hospital. But, as Neil F. Morrison in *Garden Gateway to Canada* says, surveys done by the good doctor unfortunately amounted to a wall of "insurmountable indifference" by the general public.

This did not deter the St. Alphonsus pastor. He speculated that if he could lure these religious in settling in Southwestern Ontario, he'd find the funds to build both his intended school and a hospital. His reply to the Montreal sisters prompted an earlier visit in August 1888 from Mother Bonneau, accompanied by Mother Joséphine Pâquet, who would take up the responsibility of settling in Windsor.

The city into which these sisters set foot was still primitive in many respects. It had only been months since The Great Fire that had originated in a barn near The Great Western Hotel. Both the farm building and the hotel went up in smoke. The hotel was barely two years old. Morrison says the fire also wiped out a hardware store, a law office building, the cellars of the Canadian Wine Growers Association, a jeweler's and a cabinet maker's shop. The town reeled from the devastation, but especially from the shame of the thievery that the fire precipitated. The charred remains of these establishments glared at the sisters as they made their way from the train station to St. Alphonsus Church. They would have also passed the sprawling carriage and wagon factory at Pitt Street and McDougall, and Central School, which later was turned into the town hall. The sisters on that first visit met with Archbishop Édouard-Charles Fabre of Montreal and Windsor's civic leaders for the purpose of establishing a hospital. On that occasion—August 13, 1888—the foundation was laid for the Religious Hospitallers of St. Joseph to begin working in the border cities.

On this initial trek to Windsor, Mother Pâquet, drained and wearied from the trip from Montreal and suffering from a migraine, was discomforted by the oppressive heat of the summer day as she stood there, eyeing the southeast corner of Erie and Ouellette Avenue. She stood facing the remains of a wheat field. She noted that moment in her *Annals*:

"While passing on Erie Street we saw two blacks who were mowing hay on a large vacant tract of land on the corner of Ouellette Avenue. We stopped to examine it. This place seemed to be the best we had seen amongst all of those we had visited…

We believed that the establishment of the hospital on this site would be favourable in every respect."

The sisters selected six suitable lots. Mother Pâquet scrawled into the pages of her diary that on October 10, 1888 she paid out $2,300 for these plots. She was, however, privately disappointed. She had hoped for more—she discerned the hospital needed more property, and believed it would run out of room. She also feared that those empty lots, next to her prized six, would be scooped up by someone else. Mother Pâquet reasoned there was no point arguing her case with the bishop, because he would never approve further expenditures. To that end, Mother Pâquet marched over to the adjacent properties with a shovel in one hand and a statue of St. Joseph in the other. She then buried the religious statue, placing it upside down. She then knelt in the empty lot, and prayed that God might find a way for the Religious Hospitallers to afford this piece of land. Mother Pâquet then rolled a large boulder over top the buried statue. It was not until 22 years later, in April 1910, that the sisters were able to procure those eight adjoining lots on Ouellette Avenue. Of course, by then, Mother Pâquet had already returned to Montreal where she had set about writing a history of her religious order.

Work on making the hospital, and setting out the plans for it, started in earnest in September 1888 when Mother Pâquet de-

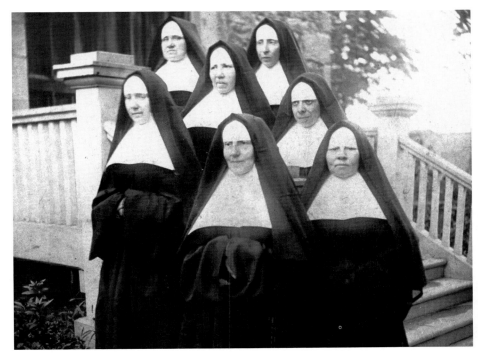

From 1888, taken in Detroit: The seven sisters in the new foundation of the Religious Hospitallers of St. Joseph. Front: Mother Pâquet

parted Montreal, this time accompanied by her French-speaking Sisters Joséphine Lamoureux, Philomène Carrière, Joséphine Boucher, and Victoire Caron. Their arrival was greeted enthusiastically by *The Michigan Catholic* newspaper in Detroit:

"The founding of a hospital in our midst, with all its attendant blessings to poor suffering humanity, seems at last to have become an accomplished fact...and under the care and management of the Sisters Hospitallers of St. Joseph—whom none are better qualified for the labor and love devolving upon hospital nurses."

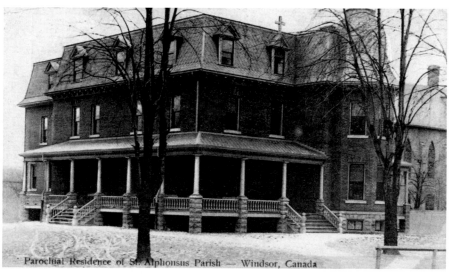

St. Alphonsus Rectory

J. Drake, dispatched six beds, a clothes closet and tables and chairs to be used in the hospital.

Still, with all the help, and the firewood to keep them cozy during a bitter winter, each of the sisters fell ill. Dr. Charles Casgrain was ushered in to help. As Mother Pâquet wryly pointed out, "God had chosen individuals who did not enjoy good health to establish this founding." The winter months were harsh, and took their toll. Mother Pâquet wrote:

"We were unable to prevent the wind from penetrating our poor apartments despite all the measures that we had taken… The wind that came through the floor was so strong at certain places that it lifted the carpeting that we had doubled in these areas…At times it was so windy in the vault that it seemed everything would come tumbling down."

Sister Rose-Marie Dufault, former archivist for the Windsor order, wrote how those first months taxed the patience and endurance of the founders: "Theirs (the sisters) was a genuine and heroic sacrifice…they never wasted a penny." *The Michigan Catholic* on September 27, 1888, described the quarters into which the sisters moved as "neither elegant nor convenient."

The sisters would reside in this barn-like building for 17 months. They survived on charity. This flowed to them partly as a result of a few small notices that appeared in the local papers. Mrs. J. H. Wilkinson, wife of Ouellette Avenue retailer who supplied shoes to the nuns, brought attention to the plight of the sisters, and asked for donations "in the way of furniture, bedding, or whatever may be useful in rendering it comfortable." A London Street (University Avenue) furniture store owner, W.

In order to warm the place, the sisters placed a large iron pot with burning embers and cinders in their dormitory.

According to Sister Cecile Comartin in *Our History of the Religious Hospitallers of St. Joseph, Windsor Ontario*, the sick were given "needed rest" in an area partitioned off in that windy, sprawling, old chapel building. But this area offered little seclusion or privacy.

Meanwhile, more funds needed to be raised. In November 1888, the sisters sponsored a bazaar that raised more than $1,000 toward a hospital. Encouraged by this, Father Wagner engaged the five in a major fundraising lottery. The sisters dutifully affixed more than 100,000 parish seals to lottery tickets that were addressed, stamped, and mailed out to the U.S. Unfortunately, the raffle had to be called off, because a new law prohibited them from operating raffles. Another venture involved collecting and re-selling used stamps, but this freed up only a couple of hundred dollars.

At one point, Father Wagner dropped off 6,000 stamps at the convent. The nuns dutifully prepared, counted and packaged these into units of 100. From the order's *Annals* in 1891, Sister Boucher, the community's secretary wrote: "We have already stated that the sale of these stamps helped to pay the interest on the aforementioned sum of money. Despite his many pursuits, this good Father spent his free time on the preparation of these stamps."

In the meantime, lacking funds and feeling tremendous stress, the sisters moved quickly to build their community in Windsor. Seven days after their arrival, Bishop Walsh came down to Windsor to officiate at the ceremony installing this new religious community in his diocese. The Irish-born Walsh, later named the archbishop of Toronto, was 37 when he was appointed Bishop of London (then called Sandwich) in 1867. He held that position for 22 years. He was a passionate supporter of the sisters, but faced the arduous task of rebuilding the nearly bankrupt diocese after the disastrous leadership of Bishop Pierre-Adolphe Pinsoneault, who was forced to resign.

So, when the sisters first landed in Windsor, they faced a cautious leader in Walsh. While urging the nuns to build a hospital, he also stressed that they needed to find the monies to finance it. Their first task was to draw up a charter to incorporate their new community in Windsor. This was done on September 26, 1888. This meant it would be independent of the Mother House in Montreal. It set out clearly their intention, which was also to receive and instruct orphans, maintain a free day school for "indigent children," but also to provide for "the relief of the poor, the sick and other needy and distressed persons."

When it came to the naming of this body, or society, it was called "The Sisters Hospitallers of the Hôtel-Dieu of St. Joseph of Windsor, Ontario." The name "St. Joseph" was chosen, oddly enough, because three of the sisters who had come to Windsor all bore the first name "Joséphine" (Mother Pâquet and Sisters Lamoureux and Boucher). This charter, approved on October 4, 1888 by Essex County Judge C. R. Horne, gave this body the freedom to act, but it also limited their access to funds from Quebec. Walsh also freed the sisters from their cloistered commitments by providing dispensation to their sequestered life. This way, they could go out into the community to serve the sick. It also meant they could venture into towns and country and "beg" for funds to

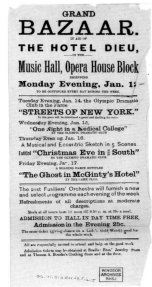

Grand Bazaar in aid of Hôtel-Dieu, January 13, 1890

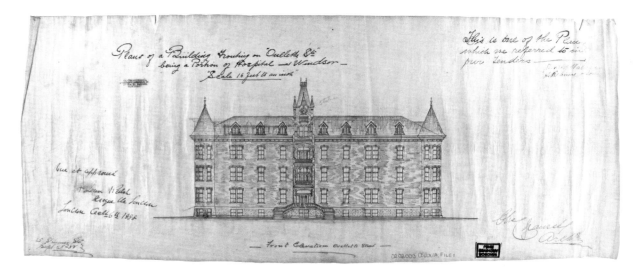

Architectural drawing of the proposed Hôtel-Dieu Hospital, 1888

build the hospital. The sisters went door-to-door seeking handouts. It was demeaning, but it helped fill the coffers. The shortage of funds, however, didn't stop the hospital construction that was estimated to reach $38,543. Work started in October 1888, a month after the sisters first arrived. The cornerstone for the new hospital was laid November 29, 1888.

Besides the solicitations at the doorsteps of residents, corporate donations started to flow in. Mother Pâquet addressed a letter to Hiram Walker & Sons on Nov. 3, 1888, thanking the company for its $500 gift. "May God bless you for this magnificent donation. In return for your kind charity our Community shall ever pray for your temporal and spiritual welfare," she wrote.

A year later, on August 1, 1889, Mother Pâquet wrote again to Hiram Walker. After all,

the whisky manufacturer by then was prospering, and had funnelled a fortune into building homes for his workers, schools, a post office, and started paving what is now Walker Road. In making a request for yet another gift, Mother Pâquet wrote: "Since Our Lord has favoured you with wealth, we are confident that you will make Him a generous return by assisting his suffering poor."

Walker never replied.

In those late days of the 19th century, however, the whisky company did help the sisters by not charging the tax on its sales of alcohol. Mother Pâquet had asked Walker about this, and arrangements were made on their behalf. Hôtel-Dieu ordered two to three gallons of liquor every three months for medicinal purposes.

The sisters never gave up asking Hiram

Walker & Sons. Much later, in 1911, the sisters were in direct correspondence with Edward Chandler Walker. The letter was addressed directly to "Willistead Manor," and thanked Hiram's son for his intended donation. He was now running the distillery. His contribution was for improvements to the hospital. The amount was never specified.

Mother Pâquet was also busy firing off letters to politicians and city officials. Some didn't respond very positively. A committee of 25 did assist her with the building arrangements. These included Wagner as treasurer. Charles Eusèbe Casgrain, an Ontario physician and Conservative member of the Senate of Canada for the Windsor division from 1887 to 1907, was appointed president. John Davis, the city's mayor, served as vice-president, M. J. Manning as second vice-president, and Edmund I. Scully, who incidentally often filled in as the altar server at the early morning mass at the convent, as secretary.

Father Wagner did his utmost in raising funds for this hospital, but his real interest was building a school for orphans of Civil War blacks. To that end, he crossed the Atlantic to bring back paintings by the great masters. These were works of art donated not just by the Vatican, but also by royalty and wealthy families in Europe.

In October 1890, *The Evening Record* reported that the priest from St. Alphonsus had amassed a collection that "as a whole is admitted by connoisseurs to be about the finest that has ever been on exhibition in this country." Father Wagner was auctioning off these works for Hôtel-Dieu at an exhibition billed as "The Windsor Art, Industrial and Agricultural Exhibition." The highlight was "Crucifixion" by Hans Memling, a 15th century painting. It was one of eight sent to the Windsor priest by the Ursuline Convent of Prague. It was valued at $1,000 "per square inch," so reported *The Evening Record*. Also included was another 15th century oil painting, "The Crowning of Mary in Heaven," by Albrecht Dürer. Other artists in this collection included such names as Reubens, Raphael, Corregio and Van Dyke. The show, however, failed to get the buyers Father Wagner needed.

Another way of the nuns raising money was in tailoring cassocks for the priests. This came about in June 1891 when Rev. Villeneuve of St. Anne's in Tecumseh visited the sisters. He was one of the leading proponents of a Catholic education, and eagerly supported the black school and orphanage. That night for dinner, Father Villeneuve brought groceries for the nuns. He also asked if the convent novices could tailor his cassocks, and promised he would encourage other priests to do the same.

Much later, in 1895—still pressed to raise funds to pay debts—the nuns found a very lucrative method of trekking to the horse races, not to gamble, but to beg patrons for handouts. This came about after caring for injured jock-

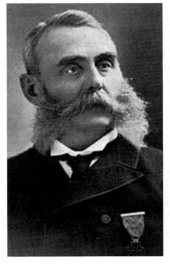

Dr. Charles Casgrain

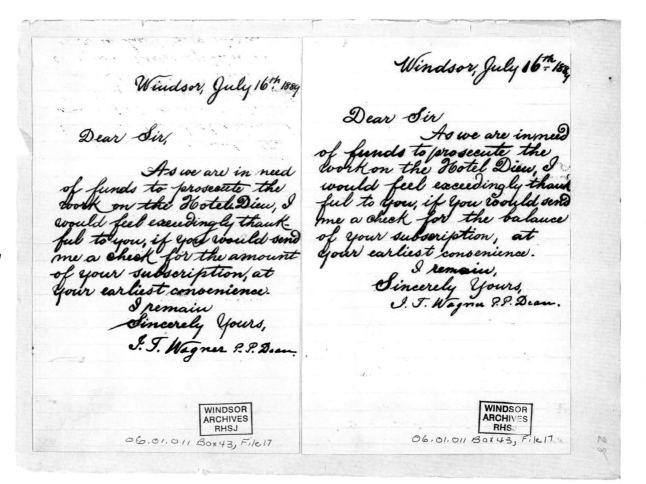

An example of J.T. Wagner requesting a donation from sponsors for the construction of Hôtel-Dieu Hospital, July 16, 1889

eys. The sisters were invited to attend a race, and told they could use an hour that had been fixed for them to ask for donations. That day they were able to collect $69 in an hour. The Racing Association also made its own attempt at raising funds, and successfully solicited more than $500, which it divided between Hôtel-Dieu and Home of the Friendless. Mother Pâ-

quet said, "This was done in order to appease those who did not see the merits of the races where so many people went to ruin themselves in order to make others wealthy…We thanked St. Joseph who must have looked after this…" She added wryly, "This was not offensive to God."

The jockeys, who had been cared for at

Hôtel-Dieu, also gathered up a small donation of their own to give to the hospital. Mother Pâquet's comment: "God allowed it to be thus for the good of our works…" Much later, the nuns were given a horse to auction off, and to that end sold hundreds of raffle tickets at 25 cents each.

On Sunday, October 13, 1889, the official blessing of Hôtel-Dieu occurred. Newspapers far and wide hailed the Windsor venture. Father Wagner, specifically, received acclaim from newspapers all over the map. *The Michigan Catholic* applauded his outreach among black orphans. Originally, this was what caught the attention of the sisters: "His purpose then was…a home for the scores of waifs of that race that can be found more numerously in Essex and the adjoining county of Kent than anywhere else in the Dominion."

The new three-turreted hospital with its Norman style architecture faced Ouellette Avenue, and was designed by Montreal architect Charles Chausée to incorporate a basement—five feet above ground—that would include a ward accommodating 30 beds, as well as a number of private rooms. In total, Hôtel-Dieu would have a capacity of 100 beds. A local contractor, Hypolite Reaume, was awarded the contract to do all the stone and brick work for Hôtel-Dieu. The stone itself was hauled by boat from Amherstburg to the foot of Ouellette Avenue. The brick came from Robinet's brickyard near Felix Avenue and sand and gravel from the nearby Pentland's gravel pit. Henry Walker, another local man, was given the carpentry contract from the nuns.

Not everything went smoothly during the construction.

The cold weather held off through the Fall, allowing workmen to lay the foundation, but construction slowed with squabbles over the carpentry. Even worse, Webster & Meath's crew of Detroit plumbers had their truck seized by Officer Drouillard of Canada Customs. The equipment they were carrying from the train station to the hospital construction site had originated in Toronto, not Detroit, and the bylaw apparently prohibited "the trafficking business" by outside teams in Windsor. These men were from Detroit. The company was then forced to hire another team, one based in Windsor to ferry the plumbing supplies to Hôtel-Dieu. The newspaper's comment: "The town people are indignant at Drouillard's action."

As for the dedication of the new hospital on October 13, 1889, it was glowingly written up by *The Michigan Catholic*:

"The sight was a glorious one…The Union Jack, the Stars and Stripes…The emerald green flag, the Tricolour waved together in the breeze…The like has perhaps never been seen before in Windsor… Fully ten thousand people had gathered at the hospital…"

That day, homilist Rev. M. P. Dowling, rector of Detroit College, opened with:

"This is a day of rejoicing for every Catholic in Windsor, and for citizens of every creed, in the whole province of Ontario because charity has built herself a home."

The hospital dedication began with a mass at St. Alphonsus at 10:30 a.m., where Bishop Walsh's address, according to *The Catholic Record* of London, Ont., brought the crowd to tears as he spoke about the "sacrifice" being made by the Montreal sisters.

Rain threatened the celebrations earlier in the morning, and later when Rev. Dowling was delivering his words to the throng, the weather turned suddenly cold. As *The Catholic Record* reported, "...the air had been chilly and sky threatening," so Rev. Dowling cut his remarks short. However, it didn't deter his flowery language as he spoke to the thousands who had gathered there:

"I see that the elements are against us and forbid me to proceed any further yet, I would not have said all that I should say if, in this brief discourse, I did not encourage you to support the house dedicated to charity today. You have planted it in our midst; let it not remain barren. Let the dew of your charity fall upon it. Let the stream of your generosity and bounty water it. Let

"...Let this house be a beacon in this city..."

this house be a beacon in this city."

The Catholic Record also lauded Windsor for building Hôtel-Dieu, and said the town was the envy of southwestern Ontario: "Streetcars, electric lights, and miles of paved roads, give the town a modern appearance."

The School and Orphanage

There is a 19th century photograph of a mission for black children in Windsor. Father Wagner is standing to one side: a stolid-looking pastor sporting a black biretta. His fat breviary is tucked tightly in the crook of his left arm, and his arms are folded. The children—five rows of them—stare glumly at the camera that has been set up in the yard.

Behind them is the wood-frame building of the first school for black children. The year is 1888. It was called "Petits Négrillons de Notre Maison de Windsor." Forty-six children were registered in that school. How this came about was the result of those early days in Windsor when Father Wagner first arrived. He used to wander through the neighbourhoods where blacks had settled. He was an eccentric creature, whose parents were German, but Father Wagner was also fluent in French, having come from the border district of Lorraine in France. He quickly acquired English in those first years in Windsor. He was surprised to find a black population in Windsor. He knew very little of why or how the town had been the terminus for fugitive slaves from the U.S. when it was embroiled in the Civil War. Wagner's chief concern was for their health and welfare. They numbered one per cent of the population in Windsor. He knew they needed a proper school and orphanage. Father Wagner soon realized they had suffered harsh discrimination, but now it was at the hands of those in Upper Canada. He acknowledged that the city offered refuge, but it didn't change the attitudes of some businesses that made it clear they were restricted to "whites only."

That's what prompted Wagner to start this mission for these Civil War refugees. That growing black population was poor, disenfranchised, alienated, and alone. From the comfortable rectory of St. Alphonsus Church, Wagner initiated a personal letter writing campaign, and dashed off thousands of petitions for donations—a mere 10 cents or more to fund his mission. By then, the Windsor priest had already started his school at the rear of St. Alphonsus Hall for the black children in his parish who were prohibited from attending white schools. Bishop Walsh responded to the news of the school with immediate moral support. On St. Patrick's Day, 1887, he wrote to the pastor: "I heartily approve your Mission among the colored people of Windsor, and I earnestly hope that a generous public will help you in its prosecution…A school for colored children is a prime necessity." The bishop also warned Father Wagner that such a school could not be

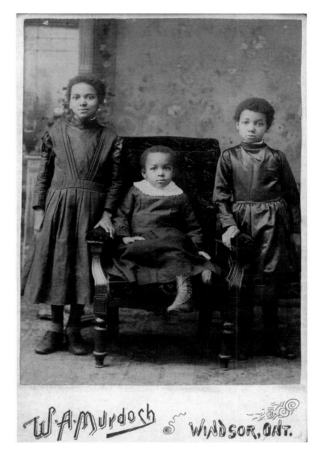

First three admitted to the orphanage in 1890, left to right, Cyrilia, Sara, and Jane Stodder. This photograph was taken by W.A. Murdoch.

carried out without sufficient resources. To that end, Bishop Walsh sent him a cheque for $50. At that point in time, Father Wagner already had 45 students in the school, 40 of whom he said were baptized.

Mother Justine Bonneau, Superior of the Religious Hospitallers of St. Joseph in Montreal, also backed the Windsor priest. Her motive in sending a small donation may have been greater—she recognized the need for a hospital, and suggested that Father Wagner might consider accepting her offer to build a religious hospital in Windsor. Father Wagner jumped at the opportunity, never pondering what this might cost. Here he was, seeking help to build an orphanage, and now he was envisioning both a school and a hospital. He agreed with Mother Bonneau to send the nuns to Windsor.

Before the Montreal sisters arrived in 1888, the Holy Names Sisters had already started a school called "Mission for Coloured Children," the one that Father Wagner was running at the back of St. Alphonsus Church. The Holy Names Sisters were assigned to these children, but the school itself lasted only a couple of months, perhaps because of the racial bias that existed in the city, maybe even among the parishioners at St. Alphonsus. It took nearly two years before the sisters of the Religious Hospitallers of St. Joseph would open the doors of the orphanage and day school in a white frame building adjacent to the hospital. Sister St. Patrice (Germaine Lussier), a bilingual teacher, was put in charge initially. She had taught 11 years at schools in Chatham, New Brunswick. Father Wagner didn't stop there. He opened up a black community centre on Goyeau, near Park Street. Out of this modest building, he provided food and clothing for the indigent black families.

The foundations for the hospital, as well as the orphanage really came together in September 1888, when Father Wagner and the sisters went through the incorporation process under the provisions of Chapter 172 of the Revised Statutes of Ontario. They formed a legal society that called itself "The Sisters Hospitallers of the Hôtel-Dieu of St. Joseph of Windsor, Ontario" for "the purposes…the reception and instruction of orphans, the maintenance of a free day school for indigent children and relief of the poor, the sick and the other needy and distressed persons."

Father Wagner was the perfect priest for this corner of Ontario. According to historian Michael Power in the *Dictionary of Canadian Biography*, he was still studying for the priesthood when he was summoned by London Bishop Pierre Adolphe Pinsoneault to begin work at the newly established Assumption College in Windsor. He taught there for three years, but, while there, also completed his theology work. In June 1860, Father Wagner was assigned to Assumption. He was barely 23. He didn't remain long. By September, he was on his way to Norfolk County, and there founded the parish of Our Lady of LaSallette, a school in Wingham, and purchased land for a parish in Simcoe. By 1865, he was back in Windsor, this time appointed as the first resident pastor of St. Alphonsus. It was toward the end of the Civil War in the U.S., and Father Wagner began visiting the neighbourhoods surrounding the parish, and was drawn to the plight among black refugees. Meanwhile, he built a rectory and also oversaw the construction of St. Mary's

Academy, a school for girls, on land adjoining the parish. By March 1868, Father Wagner found an architect to build a church that rivaled Assumption. But he needed the funds, and thought if he returned to Europe, he might find the financial support there. He actually arranged an audience with Pope Pius IX, and in Paris he met with Napoleon III. According to the *Dictionary of Canadian Biography*, both were impressed with his "determination." The Pope donated a silver ciborium, which is still housed at St. Alphonsus. Emperor Napoleon offered him a series of steel engravings. "The engravings and other donations," according to the *Dictionary of Canadian Biography*, "were eventually auctioned or sold in a series of spectacular bazaars and lotteries."

In September 1871, the cornerstone was laid for the new church in Windsor. Bishop Walsh was there to officiate. Two years later, St. Alphonsus was opened, and formally consecrated. Father Wagner and Bishop Walsh became fast friends.

But the crowning achievement for the Windsor priest was the orphanage and school that opened in 1890. As it turned out, it amounted to little because of a lack of community support. It's clear from documents from the Religious Hospitallers of St. Joseph that the sisters weren't enthusiastic about it. More specifically, the ill behaviour of the children frustrated them to no end.

A wood-frame orphanage that accommo-

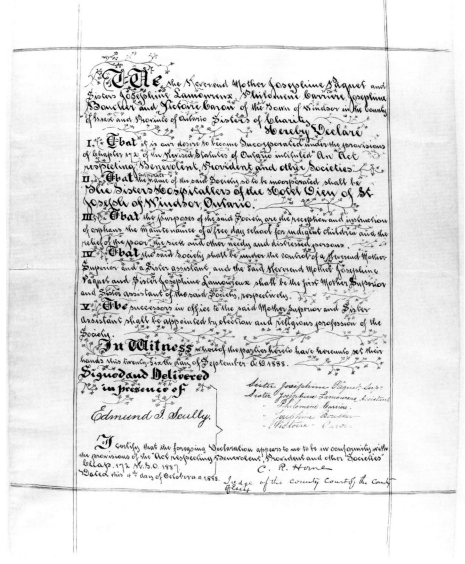

The Hôtel-Dieu Charter, October 4, 1888, signed by Edmund Scully, Secretary

dated the children was built at a cost of $4,070. It was dedicated to Saint Peter Claver who had been canonized in 1888 and declared the patron of missionary enterprises among black people for having devoted his life to helping black slaves. The school opened its doors in June 1890, and shut down March 4, 1893. From the start, there were misgivings and doubts. As reported in the community's *Annals*, those first days of running that school were hectic: "These children were, as we had been forewarned, the cast-offs of others and could not be admitted to the public schools because of their deficiency." Sister Boucher was assigned to the five black children and five orphans (four girls, one boy) who attended the first day of classes. This was on June 13, 1890.

That same week, the sisters received a surprise visitor—Hiram Walker. He wanted to become acquainted with the convent, the school and the hospital, and had already donated $500 for the construction of the building. He took a tour of the facilities, and offered assistance. He was eager to help.

Mother Pâquet knew that the success of the school and orphanage depended upon acquiring the right instructors. The Motherhouses sent her Sisters Patrice and Lachapelle from Montreal.

The happiest moment for the sisters was December 25 when Cyrilia, Sara and Jane Strodder were baptized by Rev. Gauthier, the nun's chaplain. The godparents were Senator

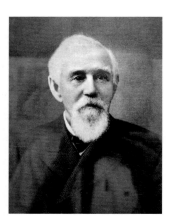

Windsor distiller Hiram Walker donated $500 toward construction.

Casgrain and his wife, F. Meloche, and Rev. Dillon and Mrs. Gauthier.

The year ahead, 1891, looked promising. The *Annals* report: "We were finally and really well established in order to carry out our mission. We were home, ready to forge on, surrounded by religious advantages…"

It wouldn't last.

In the new year, things began to spiral out of control. "The disobedience of the orphanage children…gave us worries," Mother Pâquet wrote. There were racial problems brewing too, which Father Wagner had ignored but that the sisters, who were on the front lines, had noticed. They witnessed the fierce attitudes arising among white benefactors and hospital visitors. Mother Pâquet wrote to Mother Bonneau for advice. She detailed the ruckus caused by the boys in the orphanage in a harsh indictment, calling them "rejects of the other children of their race," and saying that their only instinct was "for wrongdoing and disobedience," adding, "the girls…are not worth much more." She told Mother Bonneau, "This state of affairs cannot continue." She also predicted that whatever the children gained in the way of manners, education or religious awareness would be lost when they returned to their families. Mother Pâquet added: "It would be different if these children belonged to practicing Catholics; on the contrary, their parents are Protestant and, more than this, the majority of them allow these children to play truant every day." She then praised Sister Patrice for her work with these children: "I add once again that the teacher has to have the patience of an angel in order to sustain her task." Mother Bonneau sent an encouraging reply, but reserved judgment. She waited until she could visit the community once more.

It did not look promising. Bishop Denis O'Connor, now the newly appointed bishop of London, toured the hospital and orphanage, and openly expressed his doubts to the sisters: "As for the work with the Blacks, I will repeat that I do not see it to be possible jointly with that of the Whites." It's what the sisters wanted to hear. As a matter of fact in the *Annals*, the sisters wrote: "This...confirmed our beliefs of that moment..."

School recommenced September 10, 1891, but it was decided only to admit girls: "Along with their teacher, we did everything in our power to win them over, to make them love God and to teach them how to pray..." Meanwhile, the orphanage was in chaos: "We saw no hope of teaching them how to pray to God and the principal truths of our religion, because they would make fun of this in front of those who had been baptized, by repeating what their parents and others had told them."

In August 1892, Mother Bonneau decided to pay the community a visit. She was accompanied by Bishop O'Connor. Mother Pâquet felt her Superior was in a better position to weigh things and explain them. The bishop was also

there to bless the convent. His words moved the sisters to tears. They knelt the whole time he spoke. Afterwards, he met with Mother Pâquet and Mother Bonneau and told them their work at the school and orphanage should be discontinued, and that all efforts should be put toward the hospital. Mother Bonneau readily agreed, and when she left the next day, she took Sister Patrice with her. It was now official. The school and orphanage would be closed. Sister Carrière was given that task of shutting down the orphanage. Four young girls remained in her care. The convent decided to keep them until their parents could reclaim them. The closing was made official in a document signed December 31, 1892. The sisters wrote in their annual report:

> "Thus the project with the coloured children which had so interested us and which had caused us so many difficulties sank into oblivion. God seems to have wanted it to be thus..."

In the final report from February 1890 to December 1892, the nuns indicated that they had housed and cared for 25 children (eight boys and 17 girls) for 4,762 days for a total of 14,286 meals. Four had been baptized; six had made their First Communion and had been confirmed. In the sisters' view, according to this note in the *Annals*:

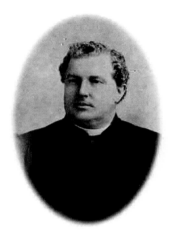

Rev. Denis O'Connor of Assumption Parish also helped the sisters out at Hôtel-Dieu.

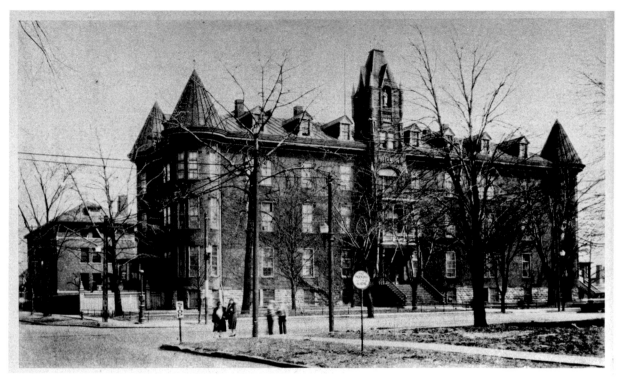

Post card showing Hôtel-Dieu Hospital, Windsor, Ontario

"If our hospital owes its existence to this laborious attempt with the black children, most assuredly it is already a very great fruit, a source of good, which is more than sufficient to reward the Reverend Father Wagner and to amply compensate us for our small sacrifices."

On March 5, 1893, the girls who had been under their care were reclaimed by their father. It is touching and revealing how the nuns describe this:

"The eldest had written to her father to come and get them as they had wanted to be able to be like the other children; that is, free to go out everywhere and to enjoy that which gives pleasure to young girls of their age, such as dressing up and make-up."

The sisters urged the girls' father to continue their instruction in Catholic schools, and he promised he would. But when the children later returned for a visit, it was evident that this had not happened. In fact, their father had the children baptized again in the Baptist Church. The nuns claimed "the bath of cold water" during that baptism caused one of the daughters,

Cyrilia, to become deathly ill. On the eve of her death, the girl's father asked the parish priest if the nuns would admit her to Hôtel-Dieu. Mother Pâquet penned a note to bring the child in as quickly as possible, but Cyrilia died. In the *Annals*, the sisters wrote that Cyrilia never forgot what she had learned. During her illness, she invoked the Blessed Virgin and recited the *Ave Maria*. In the files of the convent is also a letter that this same girl had written to the Blessed Virgin on the occasion of her First Communion May 22, 1891:

"Please pray for Mother Superior and for her dear Sisters...and send Mother Superior all the graces she needs. Send father with shoes for us, and try to send him tomorrow...Please, dear Mother, pray for Father Wagner that he may succeed in what he intended to do for the orphanage and the hospital too."—*Cyrilia*

Are they Musicians?

It was Christmas Eve 1888. The sisters scrubbed their apartments in the old Chapel. While they worked, they each promised to recite 20 rosaries, thereby saying a thousand *Ave Marias* in order to receive special graces. That afternoon, turkeys, chickens, fruit and desserts from parishioners and supporters of the hospital began to arrive. Also that day, coming in by train was a shipment of gifts from the Mother House in Montreal. The unpacking, wrote Mother Pâquet, was done with "joy and zest." Sent to them were provisions they needed, but also a bountiful share of candy, cakes, doughnuts and pictures. Sister Boucher's father also sent a crate which contained a special gift for each of the sisters. These gifts from Montreal were packed in a large piano box. The sisters had asked for meat to be sent, and the Montreal sisters packed it in between the mattresses and pillows. But when the huge box arrived, and sat on the platform of the station, Mother Pâquet wrote in her diary that people noticed the label "organ," and concluded from this that the nuns were musicians.

True Cross

In February 1889, another shipment arrived for the nuns, who were still ensconced in the weather-beaten old chapel. Mother Bonneau had returned the relic of the "True Cross" to Windsor. It had been given to Mother Pâquet upon her arrival in Windsor. She had sent it to Mother Bonneau so it could be mounted in an ornate cross that cost the convent $13. A small shrine accompanied it, containing images of various saints. "The treasure was dear to our piety," wrote Mother Pâquet. However, it raised another issue: Mother Bonneau wanted to know what was needed in the way of an altar. Mother Pâquet was tasked with providing specific measurements. "Mother Bonneau wanted to take care of this (the design) herself." The sisters sent her the height of the

"...each promised to recite 20 rosaries... saying a thousand Ave Marias..."

room where it was to be placed.

Meanwhile the "True Cross" was displayed in the dormitory in a place decorated with flowers and lit candles.

Anti-Catholic Rumblings

Not everyone was content with the Windsor hospital. That became apparent soon after Hôtel-Dieu began functioning in 1890. Jim McCollum, publisher of *The Quill*, a small local newspaper, questioned why Protestants should support a Catholic hospital. Letters appeared in *The Evening Record*, criticizing this "Roman Catholic" institution, and denouncing support for it from Windsor taxpayers. A letter signed "A Protesting Protestant" responded to *The Evening Record* in March 1893, saying the criticism was nothing more than "an attempt to bring the Hôtel-Dieu into disrepute before the public." The writer then posed the question: "What sustains the Home of the Friendless (a publicly funded institution that served the poor and homeless in Windsor)? Who conducts the religious exercises there? By whose authority? Have the Catholics growled at this use of their taxes? But one wrong does not offset another."

The Home of the Friendless' Board of Management also joined the chorus of criticism of *The Quill* letter, describing it as "scurrilous… and making a very unbecoming and untruthful attack upon Hôtel-Dieu hospital." The writer, representing the Home, went on to say that while the new hospital was distinctly Catholic,"

its outreach was not "confined to the residents of Windsor, neither to any particular race, religion or color."

The writer goes on to add:

"The whole letter shows an unworthy attempt to prejudice the minds of the people against Hôtel-Dieu and could only have emanated from a very narrowly minded person…"

Hôtel-Dieu, in fact, worked well with the community, especially the Home of the Friendless. Mother Pâquet, early on, secured an arrangement to accept patients from the Home at a specified rate of $4 per week board. However, the Hôtel-Dieu Superior was quite precise in a letter dated March 26, 1891 about the arrangement between the two institutions. She wrote to Margaret A. Black, the secretary to Home of the Friendless, and said if any patients died while in Hôtel-Dieu care, they would be buried at the expense of the committee of the Home. Mother Pâquet, interestingly, insisted that patients being sent to her must arrive "clean and neat…(with) a change of underwear."

Further clarifications followed in a subsequent letter, dated March 30, 1891, where the Mother Superior said her sisters would not be serving wine with meals to patients unless the patients themselves provided it. Neither would she accept any pregnant women from the Home, and added, "you can easily guess the

> *"Mother Pâquet insisted that patients must arrive 'clean and neat (with) a change of underwear.'"*

reason why." On the other hand, the hospital willingly accepted all the cases of contagious diseases. At the end of that letter, Mother Pâquet in an apologetic tone said, "Hoping, dear Madam, you will not be displeased with me..."

In another instance, a letter-to-the-editor of *The Evening Record* from "A Protestant Ratepayer" admonished the city's support of Home of the Friendless, and suggested that Windsor could enjoy significant savings if it simply "farmed out their charge to Hôtel-Dieu." The writer complained that the managers of the Home received a bonus from the Ontario Legislature for their work, whereas the sisters at Hôtel-Dieu "managed to increase their income—by their industry..." The letter, dated May 11, 1894, stated:

"I would have you note, Mr. Editor, that the Sisters of St. Joseph carry on their hospital at a less rate per head per day than is done at the Home; that they do not receive any grant or bonus from the city; that they are charged for their water supply."

There were many positive notices, too, during this time, notably in the French newspaper *Le Progress*. An October 30, 1890 editorial lauded Hôtel-Dieu for its "large and comfortable rooms not only for the sick persons but also for aged persons who desire board and a quiet and retired home." The article also applauded the hospital physicians, in particular

Dr. J. J. McHugh who had organized a clinic to treat patients for diseases of the eye and ear. *Le Progress* concluded:

"Hôtel-Dieu is destined...to be one of the solid institutions of the country, and therefore we consider it the duty of every inhabitant to take upon himself a share of this great work, and help by all means to make this town what it should be."

Still, the fault-finding continued. Some complained that Hôtel-Dieu wasn't paying its fair share because it had been spared municipal assessment. This was in reaction to a recent assessor's report that noted that Hôtel-Dieu wasn't on the municipal assessment, but perhaps, because it had a "convent" housed in the hospital complex, it should be taxed.

Letters soon started popping up in the papers with hospital officials vehemently arguing that its value to the community was already being realized in dollars and cents, specifically from American visitors who were crossing the river in great numbers to use the hospital. Francis Cleary, in representing Hôtel-Dieu, wrote to *The Evening Record* that these visitors were spending at the shops in the town, and some stayed overnight in hotels. Cleary contended that if the city imposed a tax on Hôtel-Dieu, it would virtually mean shutting its doors. He pointed out Catholic hospitals in Kingston and Montreal were free of municipal taxes, and

Windsor in the late 19th century had a French newspaper, Le Progres; it provided positive coverage to the development of Hôtel-Dieu.

added: "I am satisfied, Mr. Editor, that this attempt to tax Catholic institutions has not the sympathy of the vast majority of our kindly disposed Protestant fellow citizens…"

This reaction prompted one of the assessors, William Kay, on February 5, 1892 to write to *The Record*, calling Cleary's remarks "slanderous insinuations." He explained that the Hôtel-Dieu representative was concerned over a remark made to him regarding the convent determining whether a new assessment ought to be made of the hospital property.

Kay, who two years later would be named the city's first public librarian in the Ferry Street's Lambie's Hall building (what later would become the site of *The Windsor Star*), said:

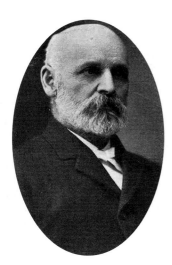

Dr. Richard Carney

"This harmless remark seemed to work up his (Cleary's) mind, like a cake of Fleischmann's yeast, though not with such sweet results, for at the first Court of Revision he quoted it against us, to my surprise, in a greatly exaggerated form, for which I, at once, corrected him. But the yeast cake kept on working, and I suspect, was the cause of the rumor which shortly before the second Court of Revision I heard was being circulated, namely, to the effect that the assessors had been influenced by the mayor."

In 1892, the nuns changed the heart of one severe critic of the hospital when it came to tax assessment. The two Ellis brothers, both lawyers, were among the staunchest advocates of taxing Hôtel-Dieu. In the spring, one of the brothers fell ill, and was admitted to the hospital. When he recovered, he conveyed to the sisters how well he had been taken care of, and that he was "more than satisfied." Following his stay, this tax lawyer told the newspapers he was "full of esteem and very grateful" to the sisters.

Other minds were changed, too, in the wave of anti-Catholic sentiment. A Protestant lawyer had emergency surgery in 1892, and was overwhelmed with gratitude to the doctors, but especially to the sisters for their care of him. Upon leaving, he remarked, "I leave, but in love with Hôtel-Dieu." This man, according to Mother Pâquet remained "devoted" to the cause of the Catholic institution: "He had many articles in the Windsor newspapers favouring our hospital…His influence in the social circles had a beneficial effect."

In another case, a patient was overcome with tears upon leaving the care of the nuns:

"I will admit to you that when I entered into this hospital, I had a mind which was much sicker than the body, and it was to convince it or to disillusion it, that I came here. For the past three days I have been observing the sisters day and night in order to discover something that I had heard and believed…I no longer believe it, and I am very angry with myself for having been so maliciously credulous. I sincerely ask for your forgiveness."

The Home of the Friendless also came to Hôtel-Dieu's defense. After yet another hostile article, one of its representatives spoke publicly about the great work of the nuns. Further to this was Dr. Richard Carney's own claims for the hospital. He was an influential area physician, having been a member of the Board of Health and the medical consultant for the Grand Trunk Railway. He also formed a famous triumvirate with Drs. Casgrain and Coventry who controlled the Conservative Party's policies in Essex County. The nuns would later name the hospital's maternity ward after his daughter.

Carney, himself a Protestant, took one complainer to task over the alleged "conversions" that were being talked about in the local papers. When one woman signed a letter to *The Quill* "A Protestant who doth Protest," Carney answered her immediately: "My dear woman, whether I am led to Heaven by you or by the Sisters of Hôtel-Dieu or by any other person, what does it matter, as long as I go there."

Despite this, conversions indeed were something these Catholic nuns did take seriously, and as part of their mission. In 1893, Mother Pâquet refers to an elderly man who died under their care, and how he had expressed the desire to become Catholic, but never followed through. To her, it was regrettable because he

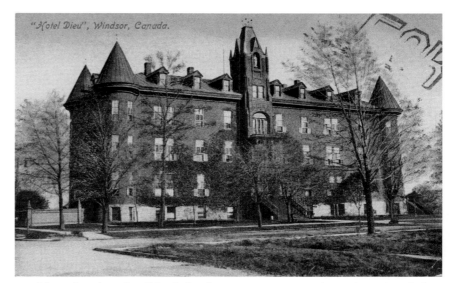

An early postcard of Hôtel-Dieu

could recite the *Ave Maria* by heart, yet never converted.

Meanwhile, Mary Elizabeth Walker, an Anglican, and married to E. C. Walker, Hiram Walker's son, was paying for magazine subscriptions for patients in 1892 at the hospital. In later years, she also took care of the burial costs and some of the hospital bills for those who could not afford them.

Perhaps the most glaring anti-Catholic sentiment blew up over the conversion and death of Colonel Arthur Rankin. This legendary Windsor figure, who served as an ensign in the Queen's Light Infantry and captured the enemy's flag in the Battle of Windsor in 1838, was also instrumental in bringing about Confederation in Canada. In addition to his military background, Rankin served as the member from Essex in the Parliament of Canada. The controversy over Rankin's death on March 13, 1893 at Hôtel-Dieu appeared three days later in *The Quill* and mysteriously, and curiously, was signed "Quo Warranto." The writer pointed out that Rankin had been given a Catholic funeral despite the fact he was a professed Protestant. The letter also accused Father Wagner, as well as the sisters at Hôtel-Dieu, of hounding him in his final moments to accept conversion to the Catholic faith.

"The surprise to me," stated the writer, "was that the gentleman in question stated a number of times during his illness, that it was his wish to die as he had lived, a Protestant, and had given instructions to the Reverend Canon Hincks (rector of All Saints Anglican Church downtown) to hold the services." The writer added:

> "He also stated to a number of leading citizens…that efforts were being made every day to induce him to renounce the Protestant faith and accept that of the Roman Catholic Church, but he steadfastly refused to do so. On the Thursday night before he died he had a relapse, and Father Wagner was hurriedly sent for, and drove with all haste to the hospital. The Colonel, however, had passed into unconsciousness, and remained so until he died, and it is therefore certain that he never accepted the doctrines that were incessantly drummed into his ears during the whole time that he was paying for medical attendance at a supposed 'Public Institution.'"

The letter writer does acknowledge that the late Mrs. Rankin, herself, had been Catholic, and that she was buried in the Catholic cemetery, but also questioned "would that reason be sufficient to totally ignore his wishes?" The letter then stated: "This single instance is sufficient to cause a Protestant of the most liberal description to see in his mind's eye, written over the portals of Hôtel-Dieu, the significant words that adorned the entrance to the ancient temple, 'He who enters here leaves hope behind.'"

The writer also described the actions of the hospital and Father Wagner as "an outrage on decency," and demonstrated "the need of a general hospital in Windsor, and that the sooner the necessity is acquired the better it will be for the community at large, as the taxpayers will be inclined to object to the paying of public money for the sole purpose of making converts to the Roman Catholic faith."

It didn't take long for Colonel Rankin's son, George, a writer, to respond. On March 20, 1893, he wrote to *The Evening Record* that this misguided story should be dropped once and for all. He said his father's "whole domestic life was so intimately associated with Catholics and Catholic institutions that he was always regarded by those who knew him best as being in close sympathy with the tenets of the Catholic faith."

Rankin also made it clear that his father in no way had been taken advantage of by Father Wagner "or the estimable staff of nurses…"

This didn't end the controversy. Five days later, another letter writer, signed simply "Citizen" in *The Quill* wrote that Rankin's case wasn't an isolated example:

"A young man named Morris, a county charge, while confined there a short time ago was repeatedly urged to become Roman Catholic and I have it from the lips of a present inmate herself, Mrs. Presious, that she was compelled to renounce the Protestant religion before she could receive any attention from the sisters in charge, and for the sake of securing peace…As a hospital, the Hôtel-Dieu does not deserve the name, as every serious case they have had has been the subject of a funeral. How could it be otherwise?

The letter writer charged that the sisters seemed far more concerned with their own religious "devotions," than the hospital's necessities, including the lack of a full-time staff physician. In concluding, the writer said that any criticism of the hospital, of course, would cause "our Roman Catholic friends (to) make a great outcry and pronounce it 'Religious Persecution' but they must bear in mind that where they use an institution for religious purposes it must be supported by their church and they have no right to expect the public at large to contribute to its support."

Despite the tension between Catholics and Protestants, many professional people didn't feel that way. Dr. Charles W. Hoare, the religious order's doctor, was a Protestant. He certainly didn't do it for the money, because when Mother Pâquet asked him for a bill he told her, "To priests, ministers, and sisters, I never charge anything for my services." As a matter of fact, for 14 years he refused even the smallest honorarium. "Such kindness warranted to be inscribed in the bottom of our hearts and warrants our sincere gratitude," wrote the sisters.

First Home for the Sisters

Their first home was St. Alphonsus Hall. It had been the parish chapel. This barn-like, wood-frame building was rough looking and chilly in winters. It faced Goyeau, and was situated on land that had once belonged to Daniel Goyeau, a cousin to Vital Ouellette. By the time the church came around to buying the property, it was owned by S. S. Macdonnell, the future mayor of Windsor. He sold it to the diocese for $1 for the purpose of building a church. The sisters moved into this old building and remained there for 17 months.

The old chapel with its white-washed walls and 25-foot ceilings is described by Mother Pâquet as "poverty personified." She also wrote, "It was dear to us because of the fond memories which were inherent in it."

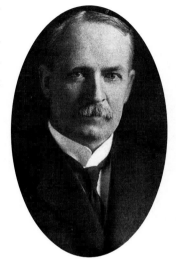

Dr. Charles W. Hoare

That first night in their new abode—the day after their arrival—was discouraging. The sisters slept on borrowed cots and straw mattresses from the convent. "Sleep was light; there was so much echo in this 25-foot high vault that even the slightest noise from outside caused reverberations thereby making a strange murmuring which took us time to become accustomed to," wrote Mother Pâquet. Yet, "even in our state of poverty, we found ourselves to be as happy as a Queen," she added.

On that second night, Father Wagner surprised Mother Pâquet with this rare give for the community's home. Mother Pâquet provided this description:

"He opened a locked drawer in his study, and handed her a silver medallion. He said, 'This is the most precious item that I possess in the world; an authentic relic of the True Cross. It was given to me a few years ago by a Cardinal in Rome. I give it to you as a gift for your future chapel.' On receiving it we fell to our knees in order to worship and kiss it…This Cross will be the guarantee of its exterior prosperity while reminding us at the same time that, if the sacrifices and the difficulties or other ordeals bind our souls to this same Cross, in return this Blessed Cross places us at the gate of Heaven…"

The sisters survived the winter, partly through the generosity of other residents who dropped off firewood and supplies. One boy stopped by the old chapel with two live chickens squawking in his grip and offered them to the nuns. That night, they roasted the birds and felt it was the best meal in a long, long time.

The sisters also kept chickens between their residence and the street in a 7-foot by 40-foot enclosure. A large box with a cover protected the birds during the winter. Here's the tale told by Sister Carrière of those chickens that provided a regular diet of eggs to the sisters:

"One night in February, 1889, during a snow storm the sisters were awakened by a distressing noise in the poultry yard, a squawking as if each chicken was being taken one by one by thieves. In great fear the sisters gave a warning signal, knocking in the windows, ringing a hard bell, this soon chased away the unwanted visitor and everything was calm again. But the next morning half of the chickens were dead, and others dying. The prints in the snow soon revealed the identity of the culprit, the 'Dog' of the Holy Names Sisters next door."

Mother Pâquet, in retrospect, was amused at the bedlam, and wrote: "It was a very comical scene to see us at work. Without being seen in the darkness, some of us went to the window in an attempt to spot the thieves. Others out

"The sisters slept on borrowed cots and straw mattresses…"

of fear dared not to move from their corners, while others rang our large bell at a window so that the Convent could hear."

The Novitiate

The growth of the religious community was needed if the hospital was going to succeed. It meant development of a novitiate. The sisters who had come here had received their early training in Montreal. Mother Pâquet sent for Sister Sophie Lachapelle. She had been with the sisters in Quebec since 1875 and acquired her training, both in the religious life, and in nursing, from working at Hôtel-Dieu Montreal. According to her biographers, she was "conscientious and compassionate to the sick confided to her care."

Sister Lachapelle arrived in the heat of summer, July 28, 1890. The Windsor community had already been operating for two years, and young women were knocking at its doors asking to be accepted. The role of training them was consigned to Sister Lachapelle.

Thus began the first novitiate at Hôtel-Dieu St. Joseph in Windsor.

But in essence, Sister Lachapelle's journey here involved training a young woman, barely 18, who accompanied her on the train to Windsor. This was Marguerite Therrien, who would become Sister Louise. She left behind her family from a small town near Montreal, and began her postulant life three days after her arrival in Windsor. Her investiture took place in October

1891. She also worked alongside Sister Lachapelle, and became the first "professed" sister from the Windsor community. Her work here was the poultry yard, caring for the chickens. She lived a rather sheltered life in the convent, however, because of deformity caused by a cancerous growth on her lip. She died at the hospital at age 76.

Even so, when Sister Lachapelle arrived, Miss Euphanie (Fanny) Ouellette was waiting in the wings. She had been under the care of Mother Pâquet till the new novice mistress came through the doors at Hôtel-Dieu. This new recruit had joined February 20, 1890, and was given the name Sister Marie. She was from Tilbury, Ontario, and had joined 17 days after Hôtel-Dieu opened.

Sister Lachapelle began working in earnest as soon as she arrived, and one by one, others started to enroll. Melvina Legault (Sister Joséphine) was the next to arrive in February 1890; and Julienne Ouellette, sister to Fanny, was admitted January 20, 1891. The first choir sister to join was Sister Eugenie Boudrias, also from Montreal. She started March 17, 1892. Lay Sister Marie Anne Therrien followed her sister, Marie Louise in August 1892.

The first candidate from Essex County to arrive was Mary McCarthy. She started March 22, 1893. She, too, became a choir sister.

Sister Lachapelle, however, couldn't remain in Windsor. She was recalled to the Motherhouse in August 1893. Later she was stationed

"The first candidate from Essex County."

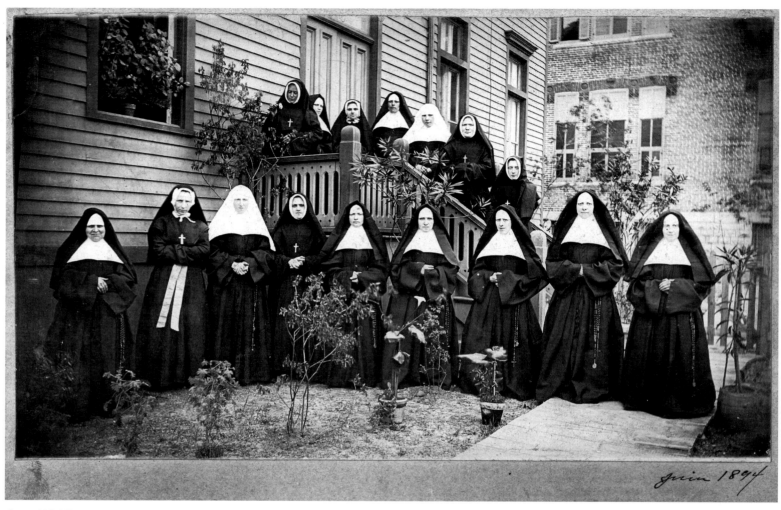

juin 1894

at the Athabaska community. She lived until she was 90.

Sister Joséphine Legault was among the oldest to enter at age 30. She was a robust woman, and her role at Hôtel-Dieu was to cook, supervise the laundry and sew. In her final years when she was wheelchair-bound, she continued to sew and prepare bandages for the hospital.

The circumstances of Sister Eugenie Boudrias, the community's first choir sister, are interesting. She was 34 when she left Montreal to join the Windsor sisters. She was obese and so self-conscious over this that she offered to compensate the community by paying a dowry of $5,000. Most young women were required to pay a dowry of $100. That was the rule, but it wasn't always followed. Many farm families couldn't afford it. At one point, Bishop Michael Fallon complained to the Windsor order that it was a pittance to be shelled out by families when their daughters were being offered such a glorious life. In her case, Sister Eugenie heralded from a wealthy Quebec family. Upon making her final vows, she bequeathed property worth more than $20,000, a sum of nearly a half million dollars today.

The life ahead of Sister Eugenie was not easy. She suffered a mental breakdown, and eventually returned to Montreal where she spent the last 26 years of her life at an asylum run by the Sisters of Providence. According to Mother Pâquet's writings, the mental disorder that Sister Eugenie suffered was the belief that she was Mother Superior. "From this," wrote Mother Pâquet, "emanated both the disagreements that she caused to occur and the pain that she brought upon herself by these hallucinations."

Life of the Postulant and Novice

The life of a postulant involved six months of training. They wore a black dress, a white bonnet and a veil. Following this, they committed themselves to a year in the novitiate, and three years of temporary vows before taking perpetual, or final, vows. The sisters rose at 5:30 a.m. and filed into the chapel for mass, followed by meditation and breakfast. Novices were assigned to duties of cleanup and kitchen work, and they sat on wooden benches and ate in the refectory at long tables. They also ate in silence after saying their Grace in Latin. The Superior would stand at the front before her own place setting, and the meal would begin only once she clapped her hands.

The day was one of work, but at 4 p.m. the sisters returned to the chapel for Vespers, followed by the evening meal. There was usually a free hour of recreation before night prayers, and sleep in a dormitory.

The Band of Five
Led by the Three Joséphines

Sister Joséphine Pâquet

She was given the name Joséphine Elodie Therese at the time of her baptism—only a few days from when she was born on October 15, 1845 in a small town about 50 km northeast of Montreal on L'Assomption River. At age seven, when her mother died, she was placed in the care of the Sisters of Providence in an orphanage in Saint Elizabeth. By the time she had made her First Communion, she was already dreaming of becoming a nun. After all, these women were her mothers—they were the ones who taught her how to say her prayers, read and write.

At 13, however, Joséphine was back at home with her father. She was there to care for her younger siblings, and remained there until she was 23. Her yearnings to return to the convent life were strong, and she finally asked her father's permission to enter. In October 1862, she had become a novice in the congregation of the Religious Hospitallers of St. Joseph. It was a natural choice. The order had been founded in Quebec—its roots and its inspiration were there. And Joséphine wanted to care for the sick and the unfortunate. It was her calling. It's what she learned from managing the family. But in those early years of her 20s, Joséphine never would have been considered the perfect choice. She did not possess that outside confidence. She is described in documents provided by the Religious Hospitallers of St. Joseph as being of "medium stature, extremely pale and frail—it was unlikely she would live a long life, let alone become a foundress."

The novitiate to her was a return to a spiritual life she had tasted as a child. She luxuriated in it, but now it was different. It meant self-sacrifice. The rigours of that life might have frightened others, but not Joséphine. The sisters wrote of her: "Nothing frightened her—work, prayer, mortifications all seemed natural to her. She was very modest, reserved and an example of punctuality so that two years of religious training gave the community satisfaction, seeing in her an elite subject."

Apparently, after she professed her first vows, she told someone that her motto had fixed itself in her resolve. "I want to be a saint," she

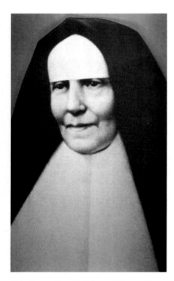

Mother Joséphine Pâquet

said. Her first job in the convent was to work in the pharmacy—this was at Hôtel-Dieu, Montreal. Her steadfast work and example soon was recognized, and Joséphine, now Sister Pâquet, became secretary for the chapter, now known as the council. She held that job for six years. As her biographer from the Religious Hospitallers of St. Joseph states, "Her well beloved Superior (Mother Bonneau) had a high esteem for her young secretary…her prudence, her discretion and thoughtfulness were unreproachable. Duty came first, and it was said her work was outstanding." While serving as secretary, Sister Pâquet compiled the 20-year history of the religious order. In the preface to what is called *The Annals*, she wrote:

"Counting on the help of God I undertook by obedience this work well above my capacity. I hope you will voluntarily forgive all that you find defective. I am happy to have done my best and I offer it as a testimony of filial attachment to my community and to each of its members."

Sister Pâquet was content to remain in Montreal. In 1888, however, Reverend Dean Wagner in Southwestern Ontario put out the word that he wanted to set up a hospital in Windsor. As the sketch of her life states, "Sister Pâquet leaving her cradle was a painful sacrifice, but she left with four companions, well qualified to help in her endeavor." On September 9,

1888, the pious sister departed Montreal, and landing here, found Windsor not at all what she had expected. Instead of a bustling and busy community that operated just outside the convent doors in Montreal, Sister Pâquet, now Superior of the Windsor order, stared "poverty, destitution and deprivations" in the face. She knew her work was cut out for her. She saw the challenge of what she called "holy poverty" as a call from God. She never once complained of life in this pioneer border town.

Instead, Mother Pâquet spoke about the progress she had been forging, but apparently she was ever aware of the financial needs of the convent, and the reality that she could not borrow, that she could not incur debt. She had an "extreme horror" of it, state her biographers.

Life at Hôtel-Dieu wasn't good for the foundress in Windsor. She resisted expansion of the hospital, fearing the lack of funds would cast the order into mounting debt. The Windsor community also resented her—the demands were too great. As a result, she decided to depart the city and return to Montreal in August 1904. But the sisters she left behind told her, "You will always be to all of us an example, a model, a stimulant and guide and especially a Mother. Are you not the creator of our little foundation and the soul of our dedication?"

The *Evening Record* the day before her departure praised her work here:

"Windsor and Essex owe a debt of grat-

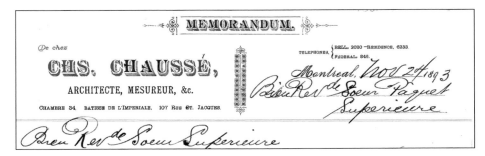

itude for the establishment in our midst one of the best equipped and appointed hospitals in the province…Her departure will be the cause of genuine regret. "

A few weeks after her return, Mother Pâquet was put in charge of novices, and a year later was named Superior of Hôtel-Dieu, Montreal. She was 72 when she died on October 17, 1917. Her biographers said that in those final moments of her life, someone close to her asked if she might offer up her "suffering" for the Windsor foundation. Her response was immediate and dramatic: "Yes, Yes."

Sister Joséphine Lamoureux

She was the second Joséphine of the three Joséphines who came to Windsor. She was 35 when she rode the train from Montreal to begin a congregation in Windsor with Mother Pâquet and three other sisters and establish a hospital here. She wasn't sure why she was chosen. She was a tall, thin woman with delicate health, but said nothing when she was asked to pack and move to a part of the country where

Charles Chaussé, an architect from Montreal, was selected by the sisters. The decision to hire him was influenced by Mother Bonneau, the Mother Superior of the Religious Hospiallers of St. Joseph at Hôtel-Dieu in Montreal. Here, Chaussé is corresponding directly with Sister Pâquet, the Mother Superior of Hôtel-Dieu in Windsor.

language would prove to be a challenge.

Joséphine Lamoureux was the tenth in a family of 11. She was born at St. Georges, Henryville, Quebec, daughter of Médard and Adèle Lamoureux. Few were surprised that she would become a nun, considering that only one of her five sisters had decided against going into the religious life. Joséphine's education was at a boarding school, but once she graduated, she remained at home to take care of her ailing mother. She was 21 when she entered the novitiate in Montreal.

Those first days in Windsor were troubling for Sister Lamoureux. Bishop John Walsh of the London Diocese, wanting desperately to build a hospital, told the sisters they would have to go door-to-door and beg for funds. He viewed this as a way of announcing to the public his intentions, and to advertise the availability of sisters to care for the sick. Bishop Walsh believed this was a need in the community that wasn't being met. The task of carrying this out was given to Sister Lamoureux, and it worried her terribly because she could neither speak nor understand English. For several weeks, she and an associate, Miss Leblanc, a tertiary of the Order of St. Francis, or a lay sister, toured the churches in Windsor and Essex County. The individual pastors provided a horse and buggy to the two. As Sister Comartin writes:

"The silent gliding figure in the rustling black habit won the esteem of many and financial support and provisions for the new hospital. The team effort of these two women was truly remarkable. After 17 years of cloistered rules and silence, she felt repugnance and fear; she knew very little English, but humbly submitted."

When the hospital was finally opened in 1890, Sister Lamoureux was appointed administrator. Like the other sisters, she rose at dawn but her task was to change the bedding, and prepare the patients for the doctors who would arrive later that morning. Her biographers state that the physicians respected her knowledge and the treatment she provided these patients: "There was a saying…'Quand on meurt avec Soeur Lamoureux, on ne meurt pas à pieds." (When you die with Sister Lamoureux, you die well.) The other skill that she developed at the hospital was extracting teeth. Because there wasn't a dentist available, that task fell to Sister Lamoureux. As time went on, Mother Pâquet started the first pharmacy for Hôtel-Dieu, and put Sister Lamoureux in charge. She soon learned her way around medicine, preparing portions in a lab-like environment before other sisters carried this medication to patients in the ward. Sister Lamoureux served as the operating room nurse, Superior Administrator (1894-1897 and 1912-1914), and much later, ran the novitiate. Sister Lamoureux—so shy and reserved in those first six months in Windsor—became the major reason for young

Sr. Joséphine Lamoureux

women entering the religious life. Finally, in 1913, Sister Lamoureux returned to Montreal. When she died at 76, she had spent nearly 56 of those years in the convent. She died at the Mother House in Montreal, and is buried in the crypt.

Sister Joséphine Boucher

She was the third Joséphine of the three who arrived in Windsor that September 1888. She was 25 when Father Wagner picked her up at the train station and drove her with the other four sisters to St. Alphonsus. She had come from one of the most honourable families in Quebec. Her father had been a prosperous merchant of musical instruments and a music master in many churches in Montreal. Her brother was a violin instructor with the Loretto Sisters in Toronto.

This Joséphine grew up under the tutelage of the Sisters of the Holy Names in Montreal. She could speak both English and French and played a number of musical instruments. Her life seemed destined for a career in music. Instead, at 22, she felt drawn to the convent. She sought out Hôtel-Dieu in Montreal. She knew instantly that's where she wanted to spend her life, helping the sick. But Joséphine was afraid to tell her father, and one night after dinner, she slipped a note under her father's plate, and fled for the cloister. Her mother was shocked. She begged her to reconsider. Her father, surprisingly, was far more accepting. On June 30, 1885, she entered the Montreal convent. She was still a novice in 1888 when she was selected by Mother Pâquet to join them on the journey to Windsor. Her biographer, Sister Comartin, said, "Well aware of the responsibilities and sacrifices she would encounter, she generously accepted. Her young heart mostly felt the separation from her family, especially her mother…"

For 14 years, Sister Boucher acted as secretary for the new congregation in Windsor. She assisted Father Wagner with the fundraising campaign, tirelessly addressing letters and affixing stamps to them. In 1890, Sister Boucher was named Assistant Administrator of the new hospital. In 1901, she was diagnosed with ovarian cancer. She returned to Montreal for consultation and refused the doctor's order for a hysterectomy. Instead, Sister Boucher prayed to Our Lady of Lourdes for a miracle. Her faith in this was strong because her sister, Emilie, had been cured that same year during a pilgrimage to Lourdes. Sister Boucher's health did improve, and soon she was back to work at the hospital. This would not last long—a mere nine months. Then surgery. Before she went into the operating room, she said, "If I die, I shall go to Heaven that much sooner. If I survive, I shall devote myself to my dear foundation." Dr. Charles Hoare performed the surgery, and Sister Boucher survived, but recovery was short-lived. She died December 29, 1902.

"Shock and grief filled the hearts of the

"If I die, I shall go to Heaven that much sooner."

novices and sisters at the loss of their beloved sister," writes Sister Comartin. "This was the first death for the Windsor community."

Sister Philomène Carrière

One of the original five who came to Windsor in September 1888, Sister Philomène Carrière did not want to leave Montreal. She was a young novice, and Mother Pâquet had good reason to bring her: she was a seamstress and could be put to good use in Windsor. One of her first jobs in the spring of 1889 was the construction of 20 mattresses. They were to be made of wool and horse hair collected from the residents of Essex County. The sisters had put out the word that this was needed, and farmers dropped off these supplies at the convent. Sometimes, the sisters collected the horse hair when they went door-to-door begging for money. On the last day of January 1890, Sister Carrière and the others moved out of their temporary lodging at St. Alphonsus to the hospital site.

Soon Sister Carrière was taking care of the orphans and school children. At night, she did the bookkeeping and helped out with the novices. The sisters who knew her best often teased Sister Carrière with being the first to inaugurate the infirmary that opened at the convent in 1891. Somehow, she had developed a "terrible swelling in her knee," and the doctor threatened to operate, but she recovered, and was back to work. A year later in 1892, Sister Carrière was appointed Assistant Administrator. In 1893, she was elevated to Chief Administrator. This lasted a year when she was re-assigned to the Motherhouse, and then dispatched to Athabaska, Quebec to set up a new foundation.

As her biographer states: "She had experienced much behind those walls (Hôtel-Dieu) and had played a part in sowing the seed that would germinate into a great hospital."

Sister Carrière was 78 when she died in August, 1939.

The Cook—Sister Victoire Caron

Sister Victoire Caron was another of the first five to make the trek from Montreal. She was eight when her mother died in Trois-Pistoles, Quebec. She was adopted by her uncle. At age 22, she entered the novitiate of the Religious Hospitallers of St. Joseph in Montreal. In 1888, she was advised by her Superior that she was being posted to Windsor. It troubled her. It troubled her even more once she arrived because she left the comfort of the convent with its spacious rooms and gleaming refectory for cramped quarters of this drafty old chapel. The conditions were "primitive" and there was little to eat. "They could only live from day to day with the help of charitable benefactors," writes Sister Comartin.

Sister Caron's role? She was the cook. For 25 years, that's what she contributed to the new congregation. "Order, neatness, ingenuity in

"Prayers to St. Joseph for a cow that would give plenty of milk were answered."

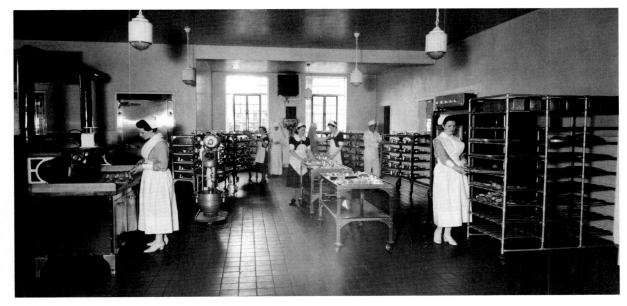

Hôtel-Dieu kitchen where Sister Victoire worked; for 25 years, she was the cook for the hospital.

preparing meals, in spite of a meager budget, characterized her life of service," said Sister Comartin, who tells the tale of whenever Sister Caron wanted something, she would place a small piece of wood around the neck of the St. Joseph statue. It would remain there until the request was fulfilled:

"Prayers to St. Joseph for a cow that would give plenty of milk were answered. A benefactor in recognition for the compassion showed by the sisters to his dying wife made a donation of $25 and a young cow. Sister rejoiced over this gift because now she could serve fresh butter, cream and milk."

Mother Pâquet, in her notes from June 1889, remarked with amusement that Sister Caron always managed to find the ways and means to feed their community in those early days: "Our dear sister, the cook, sometimes (was) accused of performing miracles at the expense of this Mighty Provider to whom she seemed to be the favourite."

In one case, Sister Caron told Mrs. Belleperche she was offering up special devotional prayers so as to secure a constant supply of milk. The woman, whose daughter eventually entered the convent, promised her a quart of milk every day.

Sister Caron remained at Hôtel-Dieu until 1913. She returned to Montreal and died of cancer in 1933. She was 72 years old.

Other Sisters from the Early Days

The Ouellette Sisters

The two women entered the convent in Windsor separately, although they were sisters from Tilbury and each knocked on the doors at St. Alphonsus Hall to speak with Mother Pâquet. Euphanie and Julienne grew up in the parish of St. Peter's in Tilbury. They perceived their future as the religious life. They entered a year apart. The two would become "extern" sisters, meaning that unlike the cloistered nuns, they could come and go from the convent. Their role was to ride horse and wagon, and go from door-to-door begging.

Sister Marie (Euphanie) eventually was appointed the purchasing agent and acted as the solicitor for Hôtel-Dieu. She also earned extra money for the hospital by visiting the homes of the sick, and consoling ailing patients for $5 or sometimes $10 per week. Her sister, Julienne, suffered an early setback in the community when she contracted typhoid. She underwent several surgeries but never fully recovered from complications.

The McCarthy Sisters

These two sisters with deep Irish roots were raised by a staunch Catholic family in Maidstone, Ontario. Mary, the eldest daughter of Richard and Catherine, was born September 26, 1863. She was drawn to the Religious Hospitallers of St. Joseph after caring for her

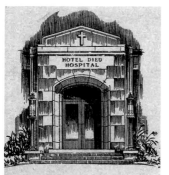

Drawing of Hôtel-Dieu Hospital entrance

bedridden mother and, after her death, for her siblings. This lasted three years, at which point she entered the convent. Mary's calling was to work among the sick. She was the first candidate from Essex County to join the community.

During the typhoid outbreak of 1896, Mary—only six months into her postulancy—was laid low with the disease, along with Mother Pâquet.

Mary trained as a nurse in Chicago in 1907 at the St. Bernard School of Nursing. She also graduated as a pharmacist, and was Hôtel-Dieu's first pharmacist. During her career with the hospital and convent, she acted as the supervisor of the operating room (OR), superintendent of nurses, mistress of novices and Assistant Superior. She died from tuberculosis August 31, 1929. She was 65.

Anna McCarthy followed her sister into the convent five months after Mary joined. She was called Sister St. Joseph. She took her final vows in October 1895. She served as Superior of the Windsor cloister from 1920 to 1923. It was through her efforts that Hôtel-Dieu was approved for standardization by the American College of Surgeons. Life, however, wasn't easy for Anna. She struggled with a hospital that was busting at the seams and growing, but whose leadership was fearful of adding more debt. There was a severe shortage of beds, and renovations were sorely needed, but there was nowhere to turn for money. Anna also suffered from lung infections, and incessant coughing to the point that she often cruised the hallways in the middle of the night in hopes of not disturbing others. She was 60 when she died on the feast of the Epiphany.

The Angel of Mercy

They called her "the angel of mercy" because of her outreach to the dying at Hôtel-Dieu. Sister Elizabeth Dupuis was on 24-hour call assisting those in the last days of their lives. This River Canard-born nun, whose parents moved to Detroit when she was a baby, would hustle from the convent to the hospital rooms, and sit with the sick. Her biographers said, "she was a friend of the people," and that she possessed that unique gift of reaching out and comforting both the dying and their families. "Charitable, submissive, zealous, always smiling and serene. The human hurts were her concern," is what the biographers said about Sister Elizabeth. She worked right up to the end. She died in 1945 from a massive heart attack. Her death was mourned by thousands who turned out to the funeral.

One mourner, a Protestant black minister, Elder C. L. Morten, is quoted as saying, "A kinder woman couldn't be found anywhere."

The Builder's Daughter

It was destined that she would become a sister. After all, both her father and grandfather—Nil Reaume and Hypolite Reaume—did the brick work on Hôtel-Dieu. The two had

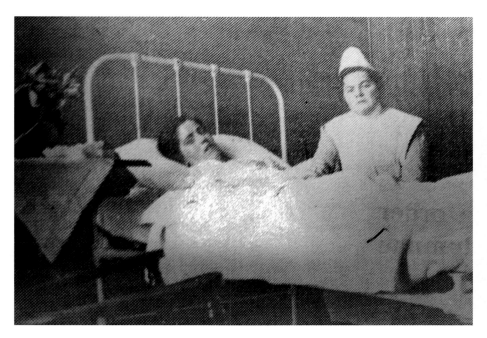

Mrs. Butts in a private room cared for by nurse Edna Renaud, 1899

become close friends of Mother Pâquet, and Angelina Reaume's father confided to the Superior that he hoped one of his daughters would join the order and serve in the hospital. His wishes were rewarded when Angelina, in December 1897, left her home at 153 Albert Road in old Ford City to become a nun. The novice mistress then was Sister Lamoureux. Angelina is described as being "a woman of sound judgment, serious, discreet, obedient…" She rose in the hierarchy of the order to become supervisor of the pharmacy, and later, the operating room. She also served as Assistant Superior, and bursar. Life proved difficult for Sister Angelina, as she came down with tuberculosis and a severe bout of typhoid fever. "She never complained, always calm, smiling, resigned and humble in the reproaches that were made because of her healthy appearance." Pneumonia was the final straw for Sister Angelina. She died at 35.

Medical Staff

In the summer of 1890, the sisters at Hôtel-Dieu drew up an arrangement with the medical staff, detailing the duties of the doctors and their authority in the Catholic hospital. The contract made it clear that the physicians would provide "free" labour to the poor. To compensate these professionals, the nuns suggested that it would enable the doctors to acquire, if they already did not possess this, "that experience in the art which makes Doctors skillful and learned, as well as distinguished…"

The contract stipulated that the poor should be attended to daily between 12 noon and 1:30 p.m., except on Sundays and Feast days. It also stipulated that the sister from the pharmacy must always accompany the doctors on these visits. The nuns, however, encouraged the attending physicians "to kindly take into consideration the smallness of means of Hôtel-Dieu and order cheap drugs, in preference to costly ones, when the same good results can be obtained."

As for other patients, who could afford the doctor, setting those fees and collecting them would be left to the attending physician. If such patients required a stay in the hospital, "board" should be collected in advance. If these involved city patients, or those sent to Hôtel-Dieu by the city, or Home of the Friendless, then the committee of the medical staff must make the arrangement for payment.

The committee—made up of surgeons and physicians—met monthly to review cases treated in the past 30 days, but also made recommendations to the administration.

The first elected officers of this committee were Senator Charles Casgrain, president, Dr. John Coventry, vice-president, Dr. J. O. Reaume, secretary, and members Dr. Onezime Langlois, Dr. Richard Carney, Dr. Raymond H. Casgrain Jr., surgeon and Dr. C. W. Hoare.

By now, 15 sisters were serving in Windsor.

The Era of the New Hospital

Construction and Layout 1890

The Norman style, three-storey, pinnacled, red-brick hospital with its mansard roof stood, as Mother Pâquet had envisioned, facing both Erie Street and Ouellette Avenue. The main entrance, however, was on Ouellette, graced by the presence of a 1,000-pound statue of St. Joseph. The basement of this handsome building with its impressive three turrets was 10-feet high, made with Anderson cut stone. The walls were four feet thick. The architect, Charles Chausse of Quebec, who charged the sisters $1,290, described the new building as "a model of strength and durability as a foundation for the present and future requirements." The

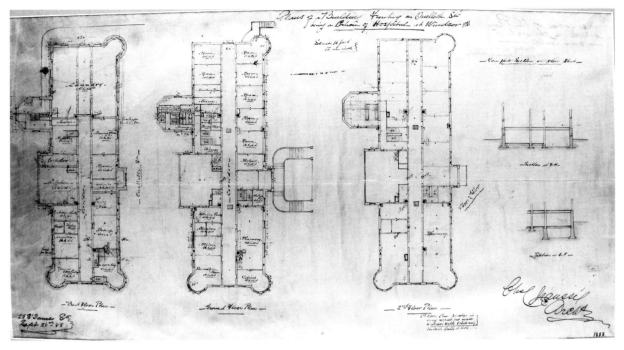

Plans for the new hospital featured 14-foot ceilings and maple wood floors.

basement was designated for laundry, ironing and baking with pantries, kitchen, refectory, laboratory, elevator, and toilets. The first floor, where the main entrance on Ouellette was situated, had 14-foot ceilings and maple wood floors.

The first floor was reserved for the parlour, pharmacy, closets, washrooms, private rooms, as well as consultation and smoking rooms. An elevator was planned for but not installed immediately; it was 1901 before it was to be placed in the building. The new facility—the architectural jewel of Windsor—provided space for approximately 30 beds. The second floor wasn't finished when the hospital opened, but the sisters had designated some of the space to be used for a temporary chapel, divided into two parts—one for the religious, the other for patients and hospital guests. Rooms for the indigent were also being planned for the second floor. The third storey with its lofty ceilings, 13-feet in height, was designated for the nuns as community rooms, dormitories and a temporary novitiate.

The nuns still planned to build a proper chapel and monastery cloister in the future. At the rear of the new building, a two-storey orphanage with a mansard roof was erected. The first floor was divided by a hall, with two classrooms—one for the boys, the other for the

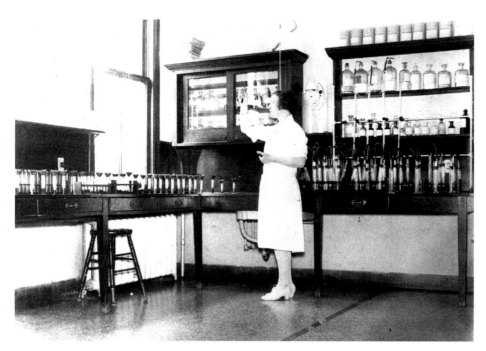

The laboratory

The first patient death at Hôtel-Dieu occurred at 7 a.m. March 8, 1890—Lawrence Costigan, a 49-year-old Maidstone farmer. The register states:

> "One of our two seriously ill patients died suddenly, but well prepared, because a heart ailment made us dread such an ending. We prayed for this soul, whose death had impressed all of the Sisters for a long time afterwards. The death was the first to occur in this hospital."

Costigan was actually the third person to be admitted to the hospital. The first patients were lodged on the first floor. The rooms had been finished there in time to receive patients. The medical problems that the nuns dealt with in those first few weeks were varied: fever, heart attack, meningitis, diabetes, gonorrhea, pneumonia, and hemorrhoids.

Hôtel-Dieu, in its 1891 annual report submitted to the government, said that it had admitted 126 patients for 1890. Eighty of those were charity cases. The hospital that year, 1891, received a grant of $1,066.25.

girls. The opposite side of the hallway included two recreation rooms, again divided for the sexes. The upper floor was designated for dorms.

The First Patients

The new hospital officially opened February 13, 1890, and boasted of potentially serving the 55,545 residents of Windsor and Essex County. Its first patient was Miss Kate Flynn. The register—*Registre des Malades Du Monastere Des Religieuses Hospitalieres de St-Joseph et des Pauvres de Hôtel-Dieu* reads: *Kate Flynn, fille de Thomas F. & Mary Mullin (Servante), (born) Irlande, (age) 35, (religion) Cath., (residence) Windsor.* She was a servant. Dr. Henry Raymond Casgrain treated her, apparently for an ulcer.

The Telephone

It seems odd to think of this in today's context, but in 1890, the pressing concern around Windsor was the need for a telephone in a few key locations. Morrison's *Gateway* noted that in March of that year, Magistrate Alexander

Bartlet and Town Clerk Stephen Lusted expressed annoyance that Town Hall was limited to a single telephone. The same situation existed at the police station. Even the police chief didn't have one. Windsor's only hospital, Hôtel-Dieu, didn't have a telephone at all. Town doctors rectified this, and rallied to have one installed there, especially following an incident in which Dr. J. A. Smith, a dentist in the old Opera House block (east of Ouellette Avenue on what was then Sandwich Street, now Riverside Drive) suffered severe burns to his face and hands when a coal oil lamp exploded in his office. If an emergency call had been possible, he might've reached Hôtel-Dieu sooner. The nuns were pleased. Mother Pâquet agreed: "Our Institution could no longer get by without one." It was installed in June 1892.

The Typewriter

Until 1896, the sisters wrote everything by hand. Ledgers, diaries, letters and annual reports all were done by pen. Scully, the hospital secretary, found a second-hand typewriter, and asked if it might be purchased. With that, Hôtel-Dieu finally entered the modern world. The typewriter cost $25. It needed repairs, but was otherwise functional. Mother Pâquet wrote, "What time this machine saved us! Even if it was used, it was still useful…" The typewriter was among "the best makes" and brand new was priced at $130.

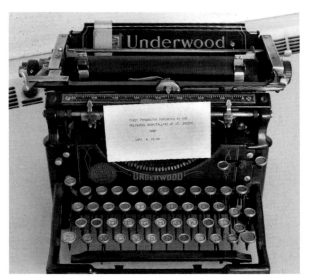

In 1898, the hospital purchased this used typewriter for $25.

"What time this machine saved us!"

The Phonograph

In January 1898, a former patient of the hospital—someone who counted himself lucky not be a Catholic—decided to gift the hospital with a little bit of frivolity. He was so thankful of the care that he had received, he wanted to do something special for the sisters. In January, he returned to the wards, but under one arm was a phonograph player. He decided the nuns, as well as the patients, could enjoy a little entertainment. He brought with him the little invention that Thomas Edison had perfected that used wax cylinders ($4\frac{1}{4}$ inches long, $2\frac{1}{4}$ inches in diameter) to play two minutes of music or entertainment, then the industry standard. The staff was exuberant, and the date was set for January 28, 1898 to play this for the first time at the hospital. It was to be played between 6:30 and 7:30 p.m. so it would not conflict with the

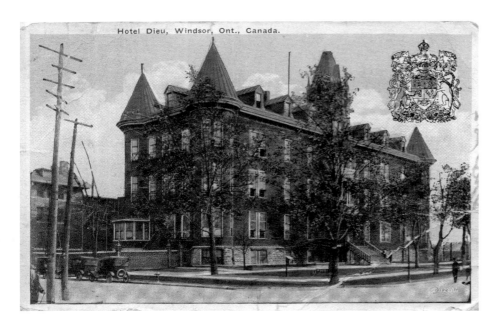

Hotel Dieu, Windsor, Ont., Canada.

An early postcard of Hôtel-Dieu after sidewalks were built

religious office or observances. However, as that date approached, it was postponed to February. Mother Pâquet's reaction in her journal is amusing, and tinged with old fashioned Catholic elitism: "We thanked this good man. Even if he was a Protestant, we had to show ourselves in favour of his wishes…inspired by an act of charity."

The Organ

Sister Hudson, who had only been with Hôtel-Dieu's novitiate briefly, made her departure in October 1901. She had donated an organ to the convent when she first arrived there, and now was embarrassed that she had decided to take it with her. It would leave the sisters without one. Arrangements were made

to send it to her, or store it. On the other hand, prayers were offered up for a way that Hôtel-Dieu could keep it.

In the midst of packing it up, Mrs. E. C. Walker stepped forward to purchase it for St. Mary's Anglican Church. She paid $220 for the organ and had it moved. But the agreement with St. Mary's was for its older harmonium to be moved to Hôtel-Dieu. The convent was delighted, and accepted the exchange.

Sidewalks, Fences, and Free Passes

In 1896, Hôtel-Dieu managed to convince the city to build sidewalks in front of the hospital. The majority of town council agreed. So did Mayor John Davis, who incidentally was Windsor's first Catholic mayor when he was elected in 1897. But in winning its petition to council, the nuns wound up having to straighten the fence along their property line. In the process, Hôtel-Dieu also built a garage for its carriages and a grain shed. It cost the nuns $2,245, a large sum for the 19th century.

Also that year, the sisters managed to negotiate with the "Electric Car" operators, or streetcar company, to use "free passes" whenever they were out visiting homes of the sick or unfortunate. This came about when Mr. Pulling, one of its employees, was hospitalized. He had been so well taken care of that he convinced the owners that the nuns should be given passes. A few days after his release from Hôtel-Dieu, the hospital's Superior received a booklet containing 100 free passes. This practice continued until 1901.

Visiting hours were never fully enforced until 1896 when a woman was fatally burned by the explosion of an oil lantern. She was admitted to the hospital, and was dying, but the chaplain turned away the woman's cousin on the advice of the sisters on duty. The relative had wanted to spend the night by her side. The feeling was, however, that the patient would last the night, and this relative should return the next day. "On learning of her death," wrote Mother Pâquet, "she reproached herself for not having spent the night and therefore publicly complained of having been sent away as being cruel."

The hospital sisters maintained the issue was "blown out of proportion by other unjust observations."

The result, however, was setting visiting hours for the first time.

The Dear Patient's Angel

It occurred on the Feast of the Holy Family, 1898. A patient who had been sent to Hôtel-Dieu by Dr. Charles Casgrain died moments after being baptized by the sisters. His name was Mr. Sicklesteil. Mother Pâquet said this patient, upon arriving at the hospital, suddenly felt "touched by grace." The doctor had sent him there "for the sake of his soul rather than his body." Mother Pâquet said at the moment he was baptized, "something strange" had occurred to him.

Meanwhile, at that very moment elsewhere in the city, Dr. Casgrain's carriage was suddenly involved in an accident that threw him to the ground. His horse broke its leg, and the carriage was damaged. The doctor dusted himself off, feeling "safe and sound," and boarded the electric car (streetcar) and continued on his way to the hospital. He went to the chapel first, and prayed a prayer of thanks for having survived this mishap.

From there, he proceeded to Mr. Sicklesteil's room, only to discover that his patient had just passed away. That's when he learned of the baptism and conversion of this Protestant friend. He told the sister on duty: "What has happened to me without causing me any serious injury is the result of the devil's hatred who wanted his vengeance upon me because of the loss of his victim. I am convinced of this."

Mother Pâquet concluded: "The dear patient's angel had therefore protected our good doctor who happily accepted the losses that he had just incurred—that of a valuable horse and an expensive carriage. He was pleased to have contributed to the salvation of a soul."

Knowing Your Place

The sisters sometimes found themselves in the most awkward and tense situations, especially when someone of higher authority took umbrage at what they perceived was disrespectful. This was the case when a parish priest arrived in town to take up residence at St. Alphonsus Church. The problem was the nuns weren't made aware of his coming.

As a result, the priest—Abbot Ferland—waited at the train station for someone to pick him up. He was advised that it would be the Hôtel-Dieu sisters, and furthermore, he would be staying at the hospital's convent. None of this the sisters knew. Feeling hurt and frustrated, he finally made his own way to the hospital. To compound things, the sisters didn't have anything ready for his arrival at their doorstep. For one, all rooms at the hospital were occupied, even the drawing room.

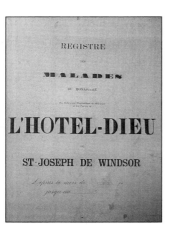
Registry of the Sick at Hôtel-Dieu

The poor sisters were forced to scurry about moving patients, and clearing out a space for Abbot Ferland. This only made him angrier, because he felt the parish priest should have tended to him. He then refused any and all help from the Hôtel-Dieu nuns. Indeed, he pouted in the tiny room assigned to him, and refused to unpack. "He stayed for eight days without wanting to empty his trunks," recounted Mother Pâquet.

Soon the bishop got into the controversy, and fired off an angry letter to the St. Alphonsus pastor. The problem was there was no room at the rectory, and so Abbot Ferland retreated back to Hôtel-Dieu, where proper accommodations were found.

It was clear the brunt of the criticism landed with the sisters—they should have known better. Or at least that was the perception of that era. Theirs was a life to serve. No wonder they signed their letters to the bishop: "Your obedient servant in Christ."

Illnesses

Diptheria and Scarlet Fever

In the summer of 1893, cases of diphtheria and scarlet fever began to crowd the hospital. The nuns tried to isolate them as best they could, but this provoked complaints from patients. Soon the newspapers were repeating them publicly. The Health Board for the city stepped in, and forbade Hôtel-Dieu from accepting any more cases. Mother Pâquet would not consent to this. Instead, she negotiated use of an empty space in the orphanage that had been closed down. Another delegation to the hospital made a visit, and decided this was still too close, even though it was 50 yards away. The visiting health group finally relented, and permitted the nuns to accommodate those stricken with the disease.

Dr. Charles Hoare's brother was among those the hospital took in. "In admitting him we made an exception to the rule and isolated him as best we could in our vacant building." Mother Pâquet wrote.

She said that when he recovered, Dr. Hoare asked for the bill, but the nuns stated they weren't charging for it. The doctor paid for it anyway. The Hôtel-Dieu Superior wrote: "We cite this deed to show the unselfishness of the good Doctor in his devotion to the community." Indeed, Dr. Hoare proved to be the backbone that Hôtel-Dieu needed. He was steeped in civic affairs, and showed leadership in the medical field in Windsor. He was named the first chair of the Board of Health, helped found the Windsor Utilities Commission, was elected mayor of Walkerville in 1917, and eventually became president of Hôtel-Dieu. He also helped create Metropolitan Hospital.

In 1894, in the midst of a flu epidemic, Mother Pâquet herself fell seriously ill. This was January, and she was leveled by a liver infection that kept her in bed for weeks. Others among the sisters, including the hospital chaplain, were also hit by the flu. This caused tremendous stress on those sisters who were healthy. Dr. Hoare worked endless hours to care for the sick. When it was all done the sisters tried to thank him personally, but also wanted to pay him. Again, Dr. Hoare refused. Mother Pâquet wrote: "We owe him a large debt of gratitude." But he refused all offers of payment.

Winter of Typhoid

William Joseph Campbell lay in his bed in "Chambre 17" attended by the nuns. In those last hours, a priest slipped in to administer last rites. Campbell was 30, and worked on the electric streetcars. Rosie, his wife whom he met and married in Ingersoll, Ontario, watched her loved one succumb in those last hours. Campbell died from typhoid. Though hospital records were specific in his case, they weren't always so accurate in others. Around him, others died from gastro-intestinal complications, influenza or fevers, when, in fact, it was later discovered, these might well have been typhoid. The scene in Windsor was grim in the winter of 1896. From December to the end of March, 122 people died of typhoid. February was the worst, with some 82 falling prey to the disease. The nuns at Hôtel-Dieu toiled most of the night, rushing up and down the dark, narrow corridors. In those years, the theory and practice of nursing was gleaned from bedside experience. It was all about caring for the ill. Nursing still clung to the model set down by its 17th century founder, Jeanne Mance, a French nurse and settler of New France. She had come to this country two years after the Ursulines had arrived in Quebec. Mance, considered one of the founders of Montreal, also established that city's first hospital, Hôtel-Dieu. From there, she provided care for the sick. She had the help of three sisters of the Religious Hospitallers of St. Joseph to carry out her mission in setting up this Montreal hospital. Windsor's Hôtel-Dieu was built on the same model, and had the same mission—caring for the sick. Nursing training by the turn of the century at Windsor's hospital was becoming far more formal; however, in essence, it still came down to "intuition," the role of comforting the sick and indigent. The young sisters were nurtured in Catholic education. It wasn't until 1919—following the First World War—that formal training was first offered at a

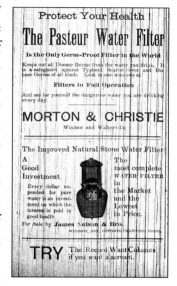

May 7, 1896. The Windsor Evening Record broke a story about the Typhoid outbreak. On the same page, there were two ads for water filters.

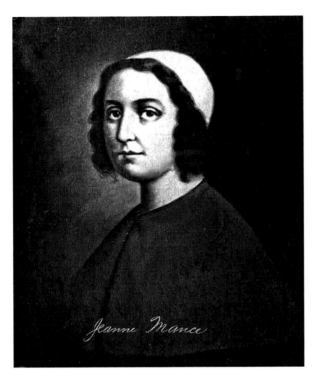

Jeanne Mance, foundress of the Religious Hospitallers of St. Joseph

post-secondary level, at the University of British Columbia. Until then, nursing skills were nurtured through the experiences passed on by midwives and from observing sick children and family. Jeanne Mance gained her own skills and understanding as a result of the absence of her parents that left her the responsibility of raising her siblings in a large family. In the throes of a typhoid outbreak in Windsor, records show no particular treatment, no medicine—merely battling back fevers and keeping patients as comfortable as possible. The culprit behind the typhoid outbreak was the water supply feeding Windsor. On the political scene, there was a war of words between Windsor and the neighbouring town of Walkerville. The two riverfront communities pointed the finger at one another. However, the crux of the problem lay with Walkerville itself. Its discharge of sewage directly into the Detroit River just above Windsor's water works intake was the source of controversy. The Provincial Board of Health finally weighed in with a 29-page, detailed study conducted in January 1896. Meanwhile, the sisters at Hôtel-Dieu were too busy to read *The Evening Record*. At one point, its editors speculated that "very little…in this cumbrous document is of much public interest." It also stated that its recommendations could not really be regarded as "advice," but as "commands." The public had no choice but to listen. The root of the controversy was hidden in an earlier investigation by local doctors who couldn't seem to agree whether the fevers and illnesses experienced by their patients were, in fact, virulent strains of typhoid. The doctors actually visited the homes of these cases and found "fair sanitary conditions." The physicians, however, did agree that impure water might have been the source of the illnesses. Other investigators dismissed the diagnosis of typhoid. Meanwhile, two doctors—Dr. Bryce and Dr. Macdonald—scooped up samples from opposite the Water Works, and one at Walkerville's intake and one at Askin's Point. The two concluded that liquid manure was "the direct and principal cause." Other investigators disagreed, especially

Walkerville authorities, including Mayor John Bott who declared the water in his town was "so clear…it is always used unfiltered," and, to date, there had been no reported incidents of typhoid. That's when he lambasted Windsor for poor filtration troubles. Others, too, noted that Sandwich did not have any incidents of typhoid. In other words, the crisis over typhoid was Windsor's alone.

Windsor, of course, wasn't buying this. Long before 1896, Dr. John Coventry, who served as mayor from 1880 to 1882, as well as the town's Medical Officer of Health, claimed the contaminants in the water originated from Walkerville—3,000 feet from the intake pipe. He said, "Refuse from cattle barns, pork-packing establishments, glucose and starch works…and other contaminants from factories…" emptied regularly into the Detroit River. He had made those remarks as mayor, and Walkerville actually showed interest in joining Windsor in a new filtration system. This was in 1887, right after the Windsor Water Works station burned to the ground. The goal was to find a common supply, situated above Walkerville. Negotiations, however, broke down, and the idea was abandoned. So, Windsor went ahead with its pump house. Still, the city wasn't about to leave its neighbour alone, and decided to take the municipality to court on a charge of "criminal nuisance" for polluting the Detroit River. In his article, *Ontario Water Quality, Public Health and the Law 1880-1930*, Jamie Benidickson said

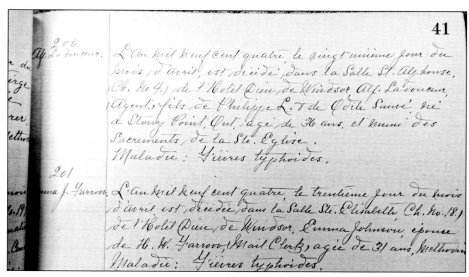

41

Typhoid is mentioned in the ledger. Two patients in rooms side by side. The ledger, of course, is written in French by the sisters from Montreal.

both communities worked out "a detailed covenant" concerning the installation of a new water intake pipe for joint use by the two municipalities. This was signed by both municipalities in April 1893. Unfortunately, it did not deter Walkerville from polluting the Detroit River.

Coventry remained Windsor's staunchest advocate, and at a hearing with the Provincial Health authorities, maintained that the Detroit River water supply was "most dangerous" and Walkerville was the culprit.

As evidence of typhoid appeared, Windsor's chairman of the Water Commission, Dr. Casgrain, took his own sampling of water on January 25, 1896, and it showed "a strong smell and tasted of manure." He said a workman from Hiram Walker reported that the sudden influx of manure was due to "the breaking of an embankment around the field where the dump

A page from the Patients' Ledger showing accounts paid in full

for companies offering water filtration devices, such as the Pasteur Water Filter by Morton & Christie. It boasted of "keeping out disease germs from the water you drink," and fighting off "Typhoid, Scarlet Fever and Disease Germs of all kinds." James Nelson & Brothers, located opposite the Crawford House, touted its Improved Natural Stone Water Filter, or "the most complete water filter in the market and the lowest in price." The company statement read: "Every dollar expended for pure water is an investment on which the interest is paid in good health."

Hôtel-Dieu was kept on alert that winter with a cadre of sisters, including novices, toiling through the night to meet the demands of ailing patients. One religious, Sister Emilie Decoteaux actually contracted typhoid while working with patients. She was ill for six weeks, but went right back to work as soon as she recovered. There was no choice—people showed up at all hours, some carrying feverish children in their arms. Others were guided through the hospital doors from the wintry night hoping to see a doctor. The wards were teeming with the sick. So were the hallways. One doctor reported to *The Evening Record*, "Everywhere you look, there was someone in need. I started at five that morning, and didn't stop till it was nearly midnight, then I went home, knowing I better get some sleep, because I'd be back again before the sun would come up."

was." Workmen quickly repaired the drainage. Some 8,000 cattle were stored during the winter on the flat fields near the distillery, and the embankment was built to prevent drainage into a large township ditch into which the main sewer of Walkerville emptied.

In that two-week winter period of 1896, typhoid cases at Hôtel-Dieu jumped from 3 to 32. Finally, in March, the Windsor Physicians and Surgeons Association agreed to the verdict over the source of the polluted river. At one point, critics of Walkerville were calling the Detroit River, "Typhoid River." Meanwhile, *The Evening Record*, while scrambling to quell widespread alarm, started running advertisements

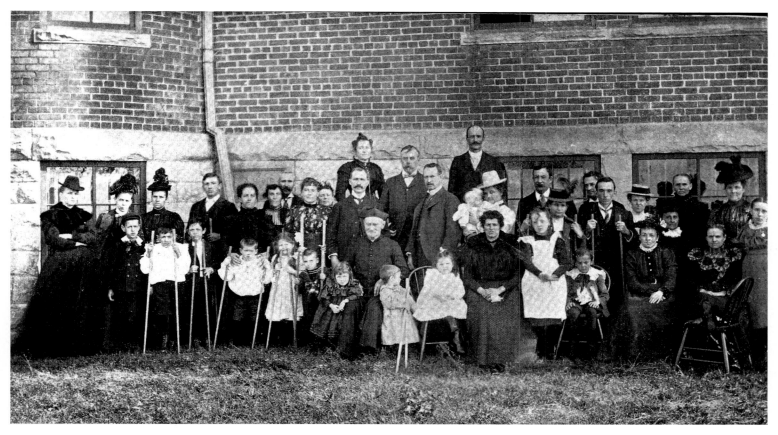

Zoé Crud—1899-1901

The sisters were keen to set up a progressive orthopedic department at the hospital, especially after reading an article published in *The Religious Week* of Montreal. The story "The Cure of the Lame" was about the Venerable Abbot Crud, "the healer priest" who was world renowned for treating infantile paralysis and diseases of the bones and joints. He operated a clinic near Lille, France, with 300 beds. Throngs were showing up at his doorstep.

Mother Pâquet, in January 1899, inquired if Crud might consider setting up such a clinic at Hôtel-Dieu. He replied a month later with a series of questions, then in July, offered his sister, Zoé Crud, a French specialist in orthopedic science. He said she could take on that role at Hôtel-Dieu. She left France with Crud's nephew, Jean, and the two arrived in Windsor in August 1899.

Crud himself set out the parameters, stressing that Mother Pâquet had to find physi-

Circa 1896. An orthopedic clinic at Hôtel-Dieu was opened in 1890 to treat bone deformities in children. Eventually this was helped by European specialist Zoé Crud. Each Friday morning this clinic would provide complete examinations and x-rays—the cost of which was sponsored by the Rotary Club of Windsor.

cians that his sister could work with. Both Dr. Reaume and Dr. Casgrain, agreed to work with Crud's sister.

Two of the staff at Hôtel-Dieu had already studied her work, and they were put in charge of the orthopedic department. Although treatments didn't begin until September 1899, on the first day that Zoé Crud landed in Windsor, a 14-year-old girl, hearing about their arrival, was presented to her. She suffered from infantile paralysis. Zoé examined her thoroughly, and began to apply her method of treatment, telling the girl she could dispense with the crutches, and maybe walk now with a cane. She had been cured. The patient "cried tears of joy," wrote Mother Pâquet.

The cure, developed by Abbot Crud, dealt with cases of congenital dislocations, as well as accidental luxation of the hip in both children and adults. Also targeted in this method were fractures, sprains, deviation of the spine, club foot, and infantile paralysis. The nuns claimed: "This wonderful treatment has contributed to the cure of thousands of lame persons, even cripples from birth."

Dr. Hoare also assisted Dr. Reaume on this first case, and remarked to Zoé, "If you cure this case, you cannot help but give yourselves good publicity." Indeed. Pictures of Harry Cotter of Windsor show the results of the Crud Method after seven weeks.

The child was paralyzed at two years old, and had no use of the right hand, and suffered a horrible deformity of the left foot. He used crutches at an early age. But after a few weeks of treatment, he was nearly cured.

The method employed consisted of massage with ointment and camphorated spirits (acquired from Hiram Walker & Sons), movement of the limbs, replacement of dislocated bones, then bandaging as required. The decision to coax the Crud family here was supported by recommendation from around the globe. The mayor of Toulouse, France wrote to Mother Pâquet praising Zoé Crud, and telling the story of his own 16-year-old daughter who had walked with a limp since she was child as a result of one leg being shorter than the other. The mayor's testimonial stated:

"In a few weeks my daughter, whose infirmity the most skillful doctors had failed to cure, was here cured of her dislocation. The atrophy of the leg, which was considerable, disappeared little by little, and today, the two legs are perfectly even…It is now three years since she was operated on."

Father Alphonse Chabot of Orleans, France, also claimed he was cured. He had been thrown from a carriage while visiting the Holy Land, and his right shoulder was dislocated: "Miss Crud so completely cured me, that I can hardly remember today which shoulder was the lame one."

Needing the financial support to continue

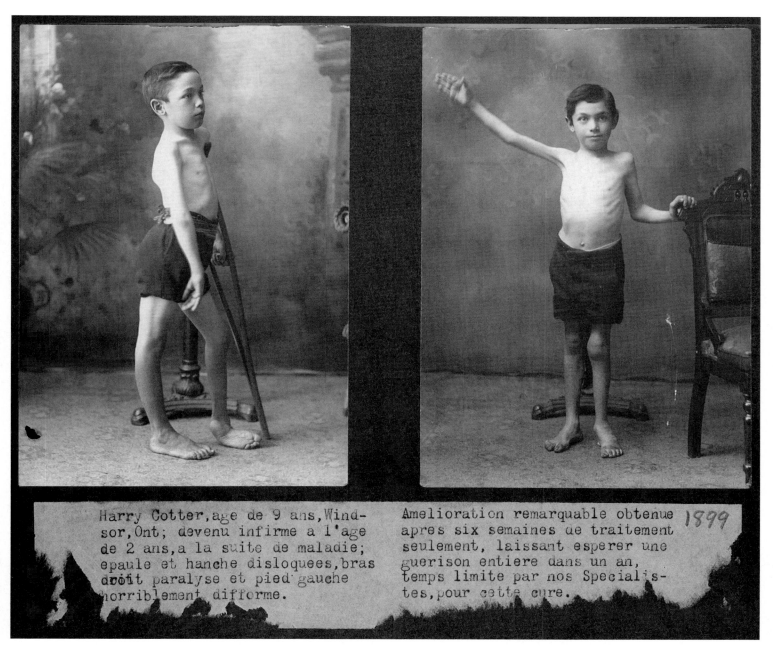

Harry Cotter, age de 9 ans, Windsor, Ont; devenu infirme a l'age de 2 ans, a la suite de maladie; epaule et hanche disloquees, bras droit paralyse et pied gauche horriblement difforme.

Amelioration remarquable obtenue apres six semaines de traitement seulement, laissant esperer une guerison entiere dans un an, temps limite par nos Specialistes, pour cette cure. 1899

Harry Cotter, age 9, Windsor, ON, an orthopedic patient of Zoé Crud with the work already being done at Hôtel-Dieu, Mother Pâquet wrote to a benefactor, T. F. Chamberlain of Toronto General Hospital, on November 24, 1899: "If you could witness the happiness and joy of these patients…you would feel deeply touched."

In a letter dated January 27, 1900, Mother Pâquet asked W. J. McKee, the Liberal representative in the Legislative Assembly of Ontario for Essex North from 1894 to 1902, for help. The response was not what she wanted to hear from the Sandwich-born politician. Criticism was leveled at the Crud method, claiming it was all smoke and mirrors, and lacked medical legitimacy.

In October 1899, the first group of patients who were under treatment were photographed with the committee overseeing this work. Other area physicians denounced the practice. They regarded the Cruds as quacks. They also said both Dr. Hoare and Dr. Reaume should quit their private practice if they were going to continue working with Zoé Crud. Preferring to keep the peace, Dr. Hoare resigned immediately. Dr. Reaume, on the other hand, stayed the course, but ever so briefly. Hôtel-Dieu suffered the severe scrutiny of medical specialists, and abuse was hurled at the hospital for engaging with practitioners whose credentials were in serious doubt. It wasn't long before Zoé made her way with her nephew and two others to Detroit. Their reception there was reserved, but after a while it became clear that people were expecting overnight success. The treatments took time. Meanwhile, as Mother Pâquet wrote, new regulations had been passed preventing "all kinds of charlatans and specialists for all types of illnesses." This new law carried severe penalties. It drove both Zoé and her cousin, Jean, back to France. In April 1901, the two bid the sisters goodbye at the convent.

Mother Pâquet maintained that the work done by the two had given hope to the mothers whose children had been afflicted by these deformities.

PART II

Growing Pains

1900-1930

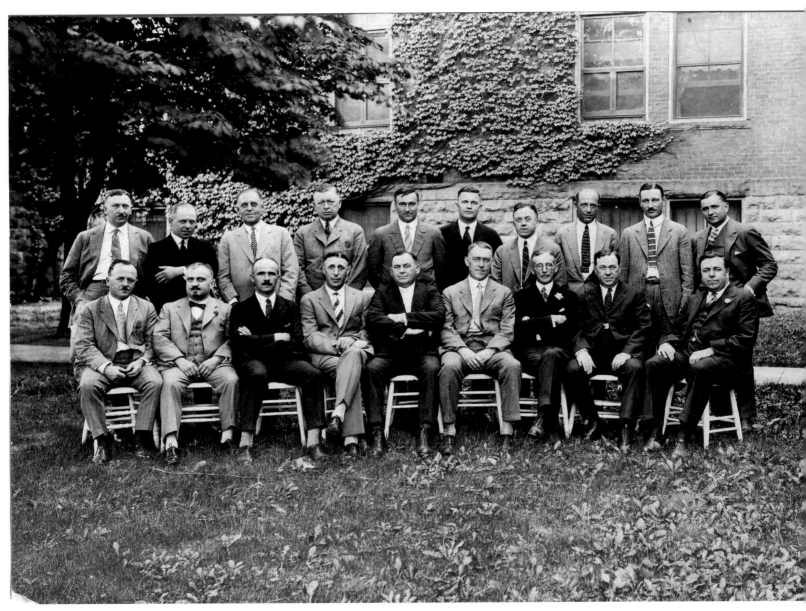

Hôtel-Dieu Medical Staff, 1925: First row: Doctors Little, Brockenshire, Stone, Campbell, White, Adams, McGavin, Moody; Second row: Doctors McCabe, St. Pierre, P. Poisson, Durocher (President), Beasley (Vice President), Crassweller (Ex-President), Dewar, Gow, Morand

Prayers Answered

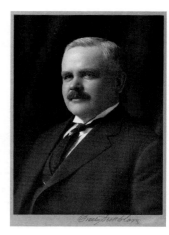

Edmund Scully, 1910, the hospital's secretary, also described himself as the convent's devoted "altar boy."

MOTHER PÂQUET'S STATUE OF ST. JOSEPH LAY BURIED IN THE EMPTY FIELD BESIDE THE HOSPITAL she had built. Her dream had been to expand the facilities. Her bishop, however, didn't see it that way, or rather didn't want the religious order, or the diocese, to be mired in yet more debt. But this was now 1910. Demands were increasing for the hospital. There was need for expansion. The property in question included Lots 7 to 14, Block 5 on the east side of Ouellette Avenue. It was owned by J. H. Whiting. Edmund Scully, the hospital's secretary, offered to buy these lots. He approached A. Whiting, brother to J. H. Whiting, and said he was prepared to pay $950 each for these parcels, but also proposed swapping some parcels of land that he owned in Detroit for those in Windsor. This offer didn't seem to interest Whiting, who wrote back and said there was an eighth lot that yet another brother owned, and the family was willing to dispose of it. Scully replied six days later on March 29, 1910: "I am prepared to pay cash…Of course you will have to pay the taxes up to the date of the sale."

Whiting's brother, who was handling the sale, said his brother, J.H., agreed to $950 for each of the eight lots, even though he felt they were "really…worth more." He dispatched a Canadian Pacific Railway telegram on March 30, 1910: *"Nine hundred fifty each lowest price considered for eight lots. A. T. Whiting, 2:45 p.m."* Scully penciled the bottom of the telegram: *Will only pay nine hundred each. Leaving for Boston Saturday.* He then wrote to Whiting, and told him he had wired him the offer to purchase, pointing out that Lot 9, immediately adjoining this property, had been sold for $750 only two years ago. Scully, in addressing Whiting, said: "I believe that you, and Mr. J. H. Whiting, are reasonable men and I think if you will investigate you will find that no one else in Windsor would make you any such offer as I have made…My offer of $900 a lot is a bona-fide one, and I have

J.M.J. ✠

..HOTEL DIEU..

Hotel Dieu, of St. Joseph.

Windsor, Ont., April 30th 1910

Alexander Black Esq.
Assessment Commissioner,
City.

Dear Sir:— We beg to notify you that we
have purchased lots Seven, eight, nine, ten,
eleven, twelve, thirteen and fourteen, block 5,
East Side of Ouellette Ave, immediately adjoining
the property we have owned for years, and
we respectfully request you henceforth, to
assess the same to the Hotel-Dieu.
By giving this matter your immediate
attention you will greatly oblige,
Very respectfully,
Sister Guevin,
Superioress.

Sister Guevin writes to the city to notify officials she has purchased more property for the hospital.

the money in the bank to back it up." Whiting countered that his brother already thought $950 was too low, and warned Scully that unless he came up, there would be no deal. The correspondence continued into April 1910 with minor squabbling over innuendos made in each others' letters. At one point, Scully wrote: "If you will state definitely what you 'will take' and not what you 'might consider' I may be able to do something. Be definite. Life is too short to be otherwise." Whiting transmitted a telegram April 4, 1910 to Boston where Scully was staying and was entirely clear about the $950. The following day, the Hôtel-Dieu's secretary responded: *Will take eight lots nine hundred fifty each. Have deeds prepared.*

Scully then wrote to Mother Guevin about the purchase, pointing out that he had agreed to $950, and that the sale was going ahead. He closed the letter in a funny but touching manner, making reference to his assistance to the nuns at their early morning masses: "Kindly remember me in your prayers… I have the honour to remain, dear Mother Superior, your humble and devoted altar boy."

Ladies Auxiliary

In 1907, a group of women stepped forward to help the sisters at Hôtel-Dieu. They saw the need for an organization that could set out independently to raise the monies necessary to augment further development of the hospital.

The Windsor Record in 1907, in commenting about this new group, stated: "There are those who realize the import and the worth of that practicable charitableness of this institution… A number of women have banded together, pledged to do whatever lies within their limited power by personal contribution and cooperation to hold up the hands of these good Sisters in their charitable mission."

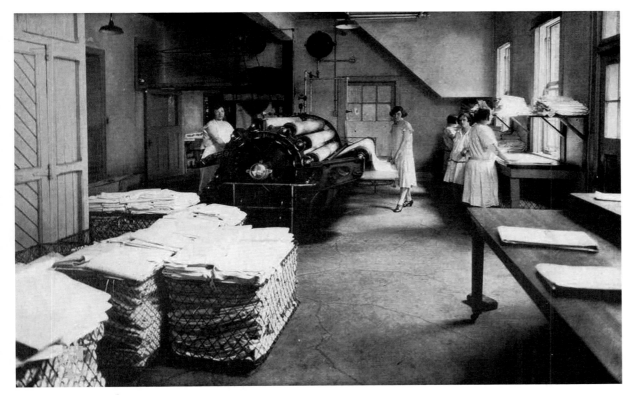

Industrial laundry equipment kept the linens and uniforms of the hospital clean.

"House Doctor," Nurses and the Nursing School

House Doctor

By 1907, clarification on the duties of both the "house doctor" and nurses was long overdue. These were set down in a memorandum from the medical staff committee. First things first: a urinalysis of each patient had to be conducted, and done soon after admittance to the hospital.

The house physician also was designated to use the hours from 1 p.m. to 3 p.m. for making laboratory examinations at the request of other physicians.

The nurses had the duty of keeping the charts of all patients in the hall desk. They were instructed, too, to keep at the ready prescription blanks for visiting physicians, and to copy these onto the patients' charts. In all cases, nurses were advised to accompany the doctors when making the rounds to see patients.

Operating room nurses were expected to set out the suitable instruments and dressings, and ensure that their own clothing and hands be "properly sterilized."

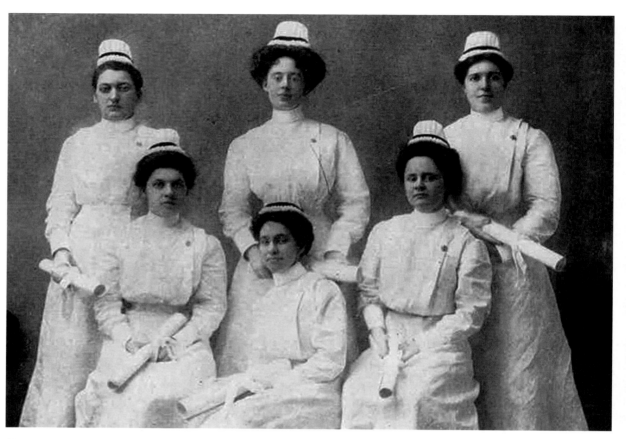

First graduating class, 1911. Top row: Sarah Wigle, Gertrude O'Donnell (Sister Adelaide), Florence Duchene. Bottom row: Olivia Welton, Mary Sheridan, Myrtle Fielder. Absent is Sister Marie de la Ferre.

Nurse's Training

The medical staff committee of Hôtel-Dieu in the summer of 1907 asked the hospital to begin an extensive three-year training program for nurses. In a letter dated August 24, a special sub-committee headed by Dr. J.S. LaBelle suggested to Dr. Hoare, then president of the Medical Staff committee, that this new training program start in October, and run until April and commence again the following October. The program or course—giving students a Registered Nurse's Diploma recognized by the province of Ontario—would cover all physical and theoretical instructions in all aspects of nursing.

The recommended curriculum would span 36 months: the first year including personal hygiene, bacteriology, psychology, medical nursing bandaging; the second year, gynecology, urinalysis, nose-ear-throat, nervous diseases; and the third, dietetics, skin care, obstetrics, ethics of nursing.

Sister LaDauversiere, Mother Superior at that time, agreed to do whatever was necessary to get such a program running at Hôtel-Dieu. The school—though established in 1907—didn't really start until 1909. By then Sister Guevin was Superior. The secretary for the medical committee wrote to her in December specifying the lecturers for that first year group. These included Dr. Ashbough teaching hygiene and Dr. LaBelle, bandaging.

The first graduation class included seven, two of whom were members of the Religious Hospitallers of St. Joseph. These were Gertrude O'Donnell (or Sister Adelaide) and Sister Marie de la Ferre, who would later become Superior of the Windsor community. The graduates in the photograph that has survived since that time are all dressed in white. Marie de la Ferre is the only one not in the picture. The following year—1912—there were only two candidates: Elizabeth Kearney and Stella Meder.

Sister Mary McCarthy, with her extensive training from the school in Chicago, was put in charge of the new school in Windsor.

"In the early years of the school, the nurses learned by doing," wrote Ada Vaughan in her history of the Hôtel-Dieu School of Nursing:

"They served in the various departments of the hospital, observing the work of each as they entered it. Formal lectures by doctors to be called at any time of the day or night were held in the small classroom or even smaller laboratory. Time on duty was 20 hours a day with 20 minute breaks for meals. And they worked! And they studied! And they absorbed nursing through every pore of their bodies! They lived in a tight little world where everything revolves around their daily tasks."

The Nurse's Duties

Nurses from 1899 and into the early 20th century were expected to care for up to 30 patients, and their duty hours were set at 7 a.m. to 10 p.m. for the day shift, or 10 p.m. to 7 a.m., for the night shift.

Besides bedside duty, or work on the wards, nurses were also required to clean fireplaces, wash stairs, sweep and dust the wards, serve the patients, wash dishes and launder soiled bandages. In applying to the nursing program at Hôtel-Dieu, candidates were asked to bring the following articles: four dresses of wash material, ten large aprons of Indian bead cotton (double-width), made with deep hem eight inches and hand gathers to meet at the back, three buttons on band; a good supply of good underclothing; a comfortable wrapper; a bag for soiled clothes; one pair of scissors; a clinical thermometer; a watch; a hypodermic syringe.

Nurses were also expected to wear noiseless low-heeled shoes. Teeth had to be "in order," according to the regulations provided to candidates. The hospital didn't want to provide

"What the angels are in God's Heaven, we should be in His beautiful world—ministering spirits and like the angels, ever bound on missions of comfort, hope and love...it became the sacred duty of the conscientious nurse to light the way to a better world..."
—Gertrude O'Donnell, Valedictorian

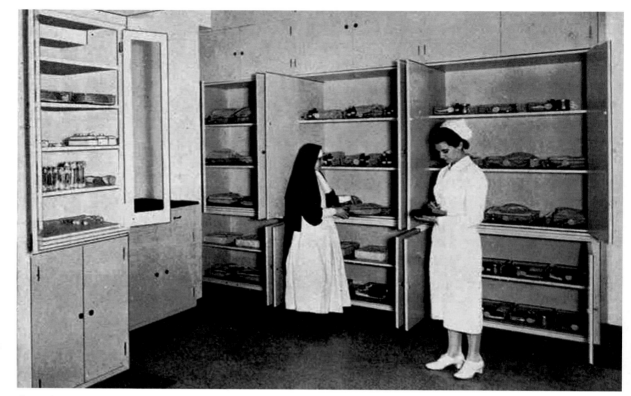

Nursing station

dental care for students who neglected to take care of their teeth.

Nurses were boarded and lodged at the expense of the hospital, but would receive no compensation. They would be expelled or discharged for negligence or misconduct. Probationary period lasted three months, after which nurses were presented with a cap. They also signed a contract at that point, good for two years and three months. Once the probationary period had been served, these candidates received a monthly allowance of three dollars in the first year, and four dollars in the second.

The Much-Touted Forgotten Item: The Elevator

There was no question that the new hospital needed an elevator. But it wasn't going to happen unless someone raised enough money to have it installed. That didn't happen as planned in the 19th century building. The sisters wanted this lift, and planned for it, and had been feverish in finding the funds to pay for other things on top of the debt that kept piling up. But an elevator? A luxury. The last item on the list. And so, installation of this modern device was postponed; at least until the spouses of the doctors took it upon themselves to raise enough to have Hôtel-Dieu equipped with a state-of-the-art lift. "Wholeheartedly, they (the wives) went to work and began to take up a collection in the city and among friends abroad," reported Mother Pâquet. The sisters had believed it was futile—they had already approached council for $500 to help build this elevator, and were turned down.

The wives, however, managed to raise enough to bring one of the first elevators to Windsor. It didn't occur until years later and required major adjustments, including digging further into the foundation to create a sub-cellar. The original contractor for the elevator was Miller and Bros., but the sisters had the architect switch to Darling and Bros., because he was tardy in getting the work done. The actual elevator was delivered to Hôtel-Dieu in May 1901, and the work began the following day. It wasn't until August 22 that a test run was done. The elevator itself cost $1,294, but its installation hiked the cost to $2,696. The wives had raised $976, including a donation of $250 from Mrs. E. C. Walker.

X-Ray

In 1908, Dr. George Chene, who grew up in Windsor but lived in Detroit, decided Hôtel-Dieu couldn't, or shouldn't, wait any longer for an x-ray machine. He took it upon himself to install one, which he operated himself. The poor doctor didn't anticipate that it would wind

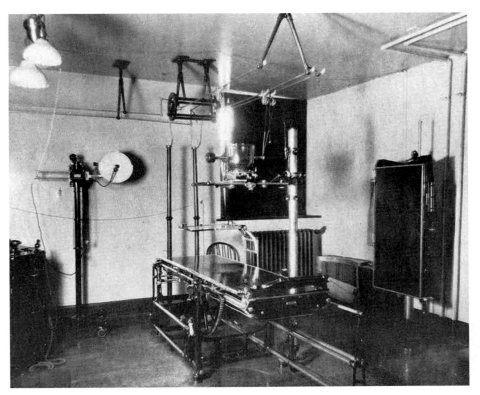

The X-ray room

up causing him even more work. So much so, in fact, that at first he spent all his time getting patients in and out of his personal clinic within the hospital—and not as much time actually doing the diagnostic work. The hospital finally had to buy its own x-ray machine in 1920.

The Laboratory

The Laboratory was opened at Hôtel-Dieu when the hospital was built. From the start, it was managed by practicing physicians of the city. Urinalysis and blood counts were done as requested by the doctors. Other exams that

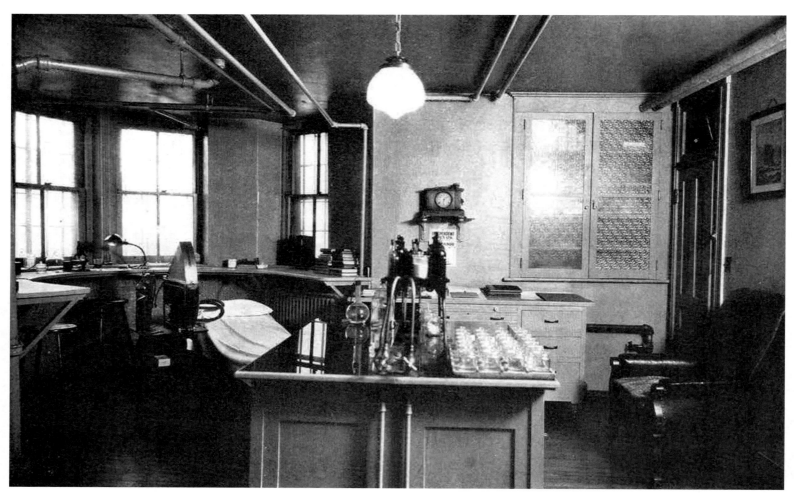

The laboratory

were required were sent to the lab in London, Ontario. By 1924, the hospital realized it needed a full-time technician. This individual was engaged in routine urinalysis that was done on all patients, as well as routine sections of all tissues removed in the operating room. Between 1924 and 1927, the lab work had increased from 2,816 exams to 6,367.

The Record Room

In 1918, the hospital adopted the American College of Surgeons' uniform method of documenting operations. In the earliest days of the hospital, the sisters wrote by pen in ledgers, and notes about patients were made by doctors. Each doctor had their own method of scribbling down notes, and filing them for

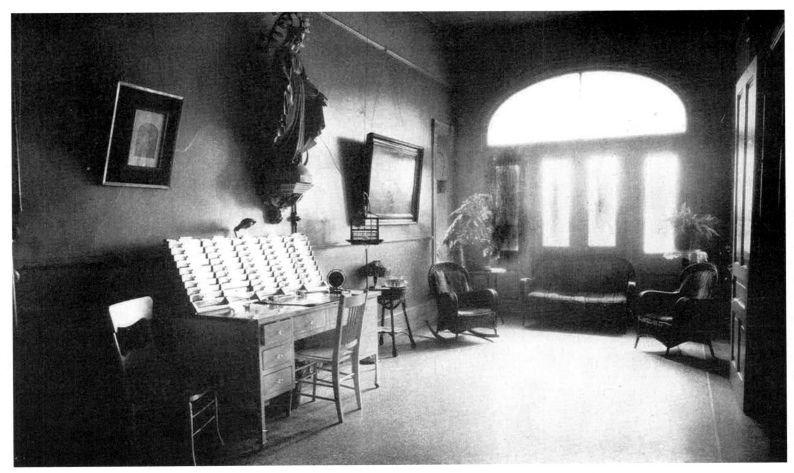

The chart room on the second floor

future use and for research work. The new system provided a means of centralizing information. As stated in *Record of Hôtel-Dieu of St. Joseph Hospital 1888-1928* the new method meant that "should a patient return to the hospital or require to go to his doctor for future treatment, the record of the former illness, and treatment (was) on file to help the doctors' memory of the case."

Some of the statistics collected by the hospital provided information such as how many patients were dealt with in a year and how many were Catholic or Protestant. For example, in 1891 the hospital took care of 126 patients whereas, in 1927, doctors and nurses tended to 3,559. In 1891 there were three surgeries, as opposed to 1,852 surgeries in 1927. Of the 126 patients admitted in 1891, 83 were Catho-

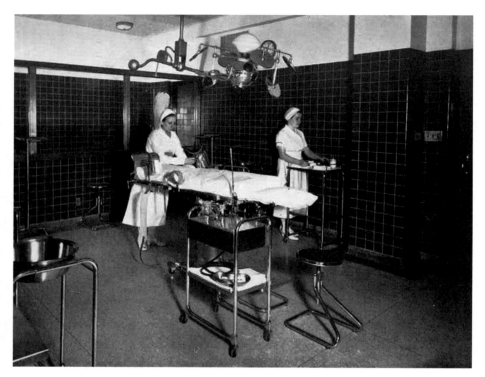

Main operating room: The first surgery at the hospital was done by Dr. Casgrain. He removed a large ovarian cyst.

transparent to ultraviolet rays) in all the windows. According to *Record of Hôtel-Dieu of St. Joseph Hospital 1888-1928*, irradiation of the infants through the glass and by the quartz lamp proved to be "exceptionally effective both as a prophylactic and a therapeutic measure," particularly treating those children confined to beds for long periods.

The Surgical Department

Room 10 on the second floor of the hospital was where surgeries were done. It had a primitive layout, and was equipped with a single homemade wooden operating table. The surgical instruments were boiled, and the dressings were sterilized on a kitchen range in the basement. Nurses carried sterile water up from the basement kitchen. Room 10 lacked a sink or even a drain, and in those early years, it was the custom to utilize large quantities of sterile water and antiseptic solutions to flush the field of operation. There was always one attendant mopping up the floor. The nuns also used a carbolic spray to disinfect the air in the room.

The first operation performed was done by Dr. H. R. Casgrain for removal of a large ovarian cyst. By the 1920s the equipment in the operating room improved, and Room 10 suddenly sprawled out to a total of four operating rooms, and one emergency room. The sisters no longer had to go to the basement for sterilizing because Mrs. A. P. Panet, president of the Ladies Aid, donated a gasoline stove. Much

lic, whereas 43 were Protestant. Charity cases numbered 80 in 1891. By 1927 the numbers rose to 660.

The Pediatric Department

The children's ward was opened in May 1927. This new development permitted nurses in training to acquire experience of working in pediatrics. The new ward was designed on the cubicle system, organizing infants and children into smaller groups to reduce the possible spread of infection. Two special features of the ward were the playroom for the older children, and the use of vita-glass (glass that is later, a proper sterilizer was introduced. It was made of zinc, surrounded by bricks, and heated by coal oil burners.

Sister Lamoureux was initially in charge of the operating room. Later, such duties fell to Sisters McCarthy, O'Donnell, then to Marie de la Ferre. In 1918, a lay person, Lillian Hannick, took over the surgical unit. She was replaced by Helen Mahoney in 1920.

The Obstetrical Department

The first baby to be born at the hospital was on St. Patrick's Day 1910. Up to that time, women delivered babies at home. Dr. J. Joinville, accompanied by Miss Florence Duchene, the hospital's first graduate nurse, delivered Hôtel-Dieu's first. The baby was Patricia Normand. Moments after she was delivered, Father Denis O'Connor baptized the little girl. At the time, Father O'Connor was the assistant at St. Alphonsus Church.

In those years, the babies were placed in baskets, and kept in the kitchen where it was warmer. By 1915, it was clear the hospital needed something better. That's when construction started, partly with the idea of creating a better obstetrical department.

His Lordship's Humble Servants— The Fallon Years

Bishop Fergus Patrick McEvay was named bishop of London in 1899. He was from Lindsay, Ontario originally and served in Kingston,

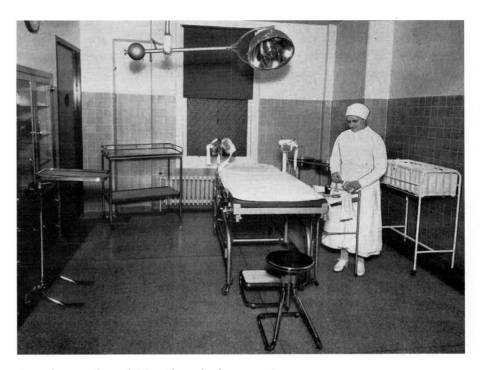

The delivery room: The first birth at Hôtel-Dieu was on St. Patrick's Day, 1910—a baby girl.

Peterborough and Hamilton before coming to Southwestern Ontario. The sisters certainly didn't mind him because, as Michael Power says in *Gather Up the Fragments: A History of the Diocese of London*, he found "ways to deal with the differences between French-speaking and English-speaking clergy and laity as Francophones sought to protect their language and culture." On the other hand, the appointment of Kingston, Ontario-born oblate priest Michael Francis Fallon brought new tensions to the diocese, in particular to the French-speaking nuns at Hôtel-Dieu. Power describes Fallon "an old style 19th century Catholic churchman," and says that he ran afoul of the

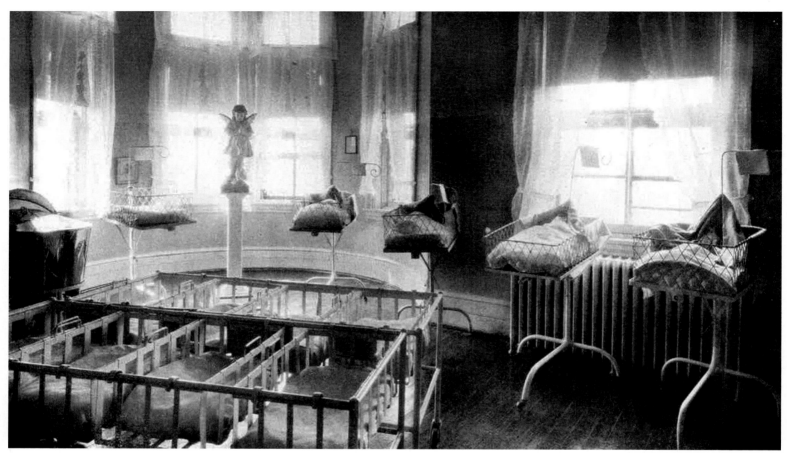

Newborn babies ward

Francophone Catholics who regarded him as part of "a conspiracy in Ontario to destroy the French language." Thus, his relations with Hôtel-Dieu in Windsor were frosty at best. The sisters didn't trust Bishop Fallon; he openly pronounced there was no future for the Religious Hospitallers of St. Joseph in Windsor. He actively sought their replacement. Power maintains Fallon's demeanor often tended to be "blunt and undiplomatic," and that he was "prone to hector his opponents into submission." He certainly tried that with the sisters at Hôtel-Dieu, but they invented ways to circumvent this. Generally, they signed their letters to him with the utmost respect and civility. Usually: "Your obedient servant in Christ…" Power's portrait of him is best summed up this way: "The public loved or loathed him, venerated or vilified him."

Sister LaDauversiere

Julia LaRose was two years old when her mother died. At first, her upbringing became the sole responsibility of her 12-year-old sister, Philomène, but soon after her maternal grandparents scooped her up to care for her. Schooling, however, was provided by the Ursuline Sisters with whom she boarded. It was because of these religious that Julia acquired a good education, including a teaching certificate. Julia briefly taught in the classroom. She owed much to the Ursulines, but instead followed her eldest sister, who had already joined the Order of the Religious Hospitallers of St. Joseph. In 1873, Julia entered the novitiate at Kingston, Ontario and, because she knew no English, found that period difficult, even "combative," as her biographers suggest. Sister LaDauversiere, as she was called, eventually was appointed mistress of novices. In 1899 she was elected Superior of the Kingston Community, and remained in that position for six years. By 1906, it was clear that Windsor's hospital needed someone of her caliber. That is what brought Sister LaDauversiere here. London Bishop Fergus Patrick McEvay specifically wanted her in Southwestern Ontario. She was elected its Superior and administrator. Her organizational skills and efforts led to the establishment of the first School of Nursing, the formation of the Ladies Auxiliary, and the expansion of three floors and a 27-bed wing. She accomplished so much in a three-year period before returning to Kingston, Ont.

Sister LaDauversiere was alive to see the first group to graduate from the school of nursing she had started. However, a year later, at age 60, the sister died.

Sister Maria Guevin

Sister Emilie Decoteaux, the maternal aunt of Maria Guevin, inspired her. It was at Sister Emilie's urging that the 20-year-old daughter of Pierre Guevin and Aurore Decoteaux would leave her home in Nicolet, Quebec, and ride the train to Ontario to enter the novitiate. As her family said, she chose to travel some 800 miles to "a strange province and a pioneer mission" to embrace a new life. She arrived in Windsor in 1897. The community of religious was still new to this part of the country. Two years after her arrival, Maria made her final vows.

Initially her main function in Windsor was to teach French to the English-speaking nuns. In 1909, fifteen years after her admittance to the order, Sister Guevin was elected Superior. It wound up being her most trying challenge, primarily because she faced the wrath of Fallon, who was causing many French-Canadian men and women to flee Ontario if they were interested in pursuing a life as a religious. The controversy surrounding the French language centred on the bishop's outspoken views regarding bilingual education in Ontario schools.

From the beginning, Sister Guevin and Bishop Fallon were at odds with one another. At the beginning of his reign as London's

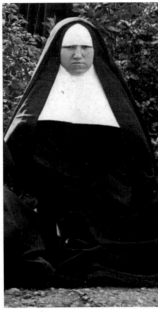

Sister LaDauversiere (Julia LaRose)

bishop, he paid a visit to the cloistered sisters in Windsor, and was alarmed at what he found. He informed them right away that he considered replacing the congregation with another that would draw more postulants to its cloister. New to this role as Superior, and ever obedient to the bishop, Sister Guevin worried over the future of the convent sisters in Windsor. She penned countless letters to Fallon. And when she stepped down as Superior in 1912, because her term had ended, Sister Guevin informed the bishop that an election had to take place. Fallon rebuffed the sister, and had this election deferred until he could find his own replacement. Sister Lamoureux was given charge—at least until a suitable candidate could be found. Bishop Fallon finally sent word to the convent and hospital that Sister St. Charles from Kingston—an Irish nun—would take over September 11, 1914. Sister Lamoureux was then ordered back to Montreal. Meanwhile, Sister Guevin remained in Windsor, there to work as mistress to the novices. She held that position off and on for a 17-year period, while also serving as secretary and councilor for the community. In 1929, she was elected Superior again, and actually received a congratulatory note from her old adversary. She held that position until 1935. It was during that period that the novitiate grew by leaps and bounds. Confidence in Sister Guevin had changed when Bishop Thomas Kidd was appointed bishop for the London Diocese in July 1931. In contrast to Fallon, he

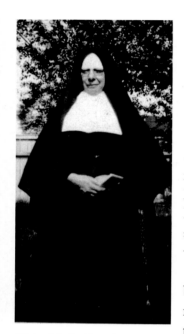

Sister Marie Guevin

was sympathetic to Francophones. When Kidd was Calgary's bishop, he took the time to learn French so that he could say the mass in French for French-speaking parishioners. He also established a French parish in that diocese. Thus his visits to the Windsor cloister were always well received. Bishop Kidd often corresponded with the sisters in French.

When Sister Guevin completed her second term as Superior, the medical staff at Hôtel-Dieu wrote a glowing letter of praise. It made up for all the doubts that existed because of Fallon's brusque handling of the congregation. After 44 years of service, Sister Guevin founded a home for seniors, called St. John Evangelist Home for the Aged. It was later renamed Villa Maria, referring to Sister Guevin's baptismal name. In the winter of 1958, 80-year-old Sister Guevin passed away. The funeral took place at Villa Maria.

Sister St. Charles (Louise O'Connor)

She was the outsider—the bishop's pick. When she arrived to take over the Religious Hospitallers of St. Joseph in Windsor, the community silently accepted her. After all, though she was from the same religious order, she had come from the Kingston congregation, not Quebec. The majority of those in Windsor were French-speaking. Even the girls being encouraged to join were from neighbouring French-speaking communities like St. Joachim, Pointe-aux-Roches and Pain Court. Sister St.

Charles didn't know a word of French. She was named Superior in September 1914. Bishop Fallon also named Maidstone-born Annie McCarthy (Sister St. Joseph) as assistant and Sister O'Donnell as hospital administrator. These three English-speaking nuns were now in charge of the convent in Windsor that was predominantly French. Sister St. Charles also ran the hospital.

She was educated by the Loretto Sisters of Toronto, entered the Religious Hospitallers of St. Joseph in Kingston, and was the sister of the Irish Senator, Frank O'Connor, a good friend of Fallon. Sister St. Charles spent three years as Superior and administrator of Hôtel-Dieu, and during that time established the obstetrical department (1915) and organized the 25th anniversary celebrations of the order's presence in Windsor. Though her appointment was controversial in a way, this English-speaking Mother Superior was a prudent choice on the part of Bishop Fallon. She certainly had experience and knowledge. Long before coming to Windsor, she had been sent to Chicago to study nursing school administration from the St. Bernard School of Nursing, enabling her to establish a School of Nursing in 1912 as part of the Kingston congregation.

While she was in Windsor, Sister St. Charles also commissioned detailed plans for a new residence and a chapel both of which were finally constructed in 1919. She is described by her hospital archivists as being "a woman of self-sacrifice and courage." On the other hand, within five months after her arrival here, she might have startled other pious sisters when she put in an order to Jacques and Brooke, a local furniture company, to furnish her private room in the cloister. She ordered a new bed, a set of pillows and pillowcases, sheets, blankets, two rugs, curtains, a bureau, a desk and a rocking chair. It totaled $105.55.

Sister St. Charles didn't stay in Windsor long. By 1917, she was back in Kingston, and died there in September of that year. At the time of her death, *The Kingston Whig* described this Irish sister as "heroic in the discharge of her duty." The writer went on to state that her choice by Bishop Fallon proved to be what Windsor needed most because when she arrived at Hôtel-Dieu, she found it to be "far short of the demand from the public and required thoroughly experienced women to build and renovate." The article goes on to say that while Sister St. Charles was in Windsor, "she won all the hearts and soothed all ills, thus fulfilling the duties of a perfect hospitaller."

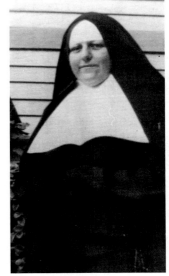

Sister St. Charles
(Louise O'Connor)

Sister Cecile Belleperche

Cecile Belleperche grew up in the parish of Notre Dame du Lac, commonly known around Windsor as Holy Rosary Parish, a building that now stands empty facing the Detroit River in old Ford City. She succeeded Mother St. Charles in 1917 as Superior of Hôtel-Dieu.

But the journey to the convent wasn't always easy. When she was 16, and attending St. Mary's Academy, she fell ill and was forced to return to the farm. However, she did not relinquish her dream of a religious life. Under the guidance of Mother Pâquet, and her assistant, Sister Lamoureux, she found herself drawn to the convent life and the work at the hospital. Cecile started in the novitiate in June 1900. At the time, she wrote, "Our canonical novitiate was not as severe as today, due to the Christian education received in our families. The formation was more practical than theological: there were fewer conferences and studies but more beneficial examples."

By 1907, Hôtel-Dieu had its own School of Nursing, and Sister Belleperche's sister, Eugenie Belleperche, was the first superintendent. The two helped in the formation of lay nurses. With the advent of Bishop Fallon's interference in the convent, Sister Belleperche was assigned to managing the novices. She did this for three years. In 1917, she was elected Superior. She saw this as a challenge, especially because the convent's numbers had been seriously depleted over the past 12 years. Some of this was due to Fallon's influence, and the pressure he brought to the convent. The fact was that some candidates—for one reason or another—had been denied at the point of admission. The future of Hôtel-Dieu was in doubt, and the responsibility for changing that fell to the first Essex County-born Superior of the order. Within a few months of her election as Mother Superior on

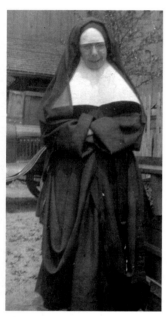

Sister Cecile Belleperche

September 10, 1917, Sister Belleperche wrote to Fallon, advising him that she was quitting. The London bishop was in Baltimore leading a retreat of priests in that archdiocese, and replied that he would deal with the request when he returned. He also told Sister Belleperche that it was now "clear" to him that her religious order could no longer continue in Windsor, and needed to be replaced by one that could handle the demands. He wrote: "Hôtel-Dieu Hospital…should pass into the charge of some community sufficiently numerous to meet the needs of the situation."

He also chastised the nuns in Windsor for their utter failure in proper "observance of the Rule of religious life," and accused the Superior of abdicating all duties in making sure the rules were enforced. He also denied her request. The matter doesn't end there. Ten days later when Fallon was in Washington, D.C., he reiterated the need for the nuns to pack up and leave Windsor. The bishop wrote:

"I must point out to you that there is simply no hope for the future of your community in Windsor unless two results can be reached. They are the revival of the spiritual and practice of religious observance, and the obtaining of postulants whose character and disposition will assure fitting subjects for the future."

Sister Belleperche pursued the matter further. She petitioned Fallon to relieve her of her position. He refused again, and in a letter dated November 7, 1917, said:

"I am very anxious over your letters of Oct. 18 and Nov. 5 in which you urge me to relieve you of your duties of Superior for your community. I should feel inclined to meet your wishes were it not for the following reasons: a) you have been only four months Superior. It does not seem a long enough time to give matters a fair trial; b) So far as the other sisters are concerned, you are their duly elected choice, and as you say, 'they should put up with the consequences;' c) If I accept your resignation things will be worse than ever. There is no other sister better able than you to do the duty of the office of Superior."

Sister Belleperche scrawled out a frustrated response at the bottom of his letter, and never sent it, but it remains there for historians in the archives of the Religious Hospitallers of St. Joseph: "Do you think there is any use in sending in my resignation? After the tone of this letter!"

If this tug-of-war with the bishop wasn't enough, the Religious Hospitallers in Windsor, under Sister Belleperche, were further chastised for failing to round up an altar server for their early morning mass at 6 a.m. Fallon dashed off a response May 22, 1919 stating that the sisters were prohibited from being altar servers. "It ought never to be impossible to find a server in Windsor," Fallon countered, ordering the sisters to make "further zealous efforts."

Sister Belleperche continued in spite of personal health problems and Fallon's bullying. One of her positive moves as Superior was to have Hôtel-Dieu join the American Catholic Hospital Association. She also opened up new convent quarters with a new chapel. As well, she shepherded the hospital through the 1918 Spanish Flu epidemic when the institution's rooms and corridors were jammed with patients.

When Sister Belleperche finally stepped down as Superior in 1920, she was appointed Assistant Superior, a post she managed to keep until 1925. She also served the hospital as its bursar, annalist, medical archivist and librarian. Sister Belleperche also organized the medical records for the hospital. A provincial inspector later remarked that her work in preparing these documents was the best he had ever seen. The last 18 months of Sister Belleperche's life were spent battling cancer. Notes that she left behind summed up her vocation: "My greatest desire was the spiritual and temporal prosperity of the community, especially the novitiate. We can never do too much for our community, the Church, and for God. Selfishness is a mark of tepidity, the ruin of fraternal charity and of religious life." Sister Belleperche died at 59. She is buried in St. Alphonsus Cemetery in Windsor.

"...There is simply no hope for the future of your community in Windsor..."
— Bishop Fallon to the Hôtel-Dieu Sisters

Sister St. Joseph

Anna McCarthy, known as Sister St. Joseph, followed Sister Belleperche as Mother Superior. She was from Maidstone, Ontario, the daughter of Richard McCarthy and Catherine McCann. She attended Essex High School, and worked for her father on the farm. Her eldest sister, Mary, joined the Religious Hospitallers of Windsor five months before Anna decided to enter in August 1893. She was 25. Anna was destined for the convent. But health problems plagued her time at Hôtel-Dieu. She endured severe insomnia and coughed incessantly due to lung problems. Still, she was always the first at meditation at 4:30 a.m. She rarely—if ever—complained. She devoted herself to the care of others. She became Superior in 1920 and held that position for three years. "Of delicate constitution, but strong of will, strengthened by God's grace, this enabled her to bear the difficulties of that position," write the sisters. "Many problems were encountered; the hospital was too small; there were shortages of beds; renovations of departments were needed; finance was lacking." During those three years, Sister St. Joseph—afflicted by continual physical suffering—managed to carry out her duties, and was loved by the patients she attended.

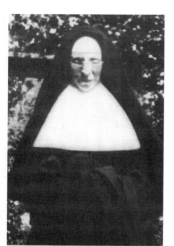

Sister St. Joseph (Anna McCarthy)

Sister Marie de la Ferre

Laura LeBoeuf was another from Quebec, hailing from St. Jean Deschallions. In 1900, at age 14, her parents moved to St. Joachim. Six years later, Laura joined the sisters at Hôtel-Dieu. She was the third of four sisters to enter religious life. In November 1908, she made her vows. She also enrolled in the first class of formal training at Hôtel-Dieu's new school of nursing. She struggled in the beginning because she spoke not a word of English. In 1911, Sister Marie was among the graduating class.

Sister Marie's involvement in Hôtel-Dieu ran deep. She was supervisor in various departments, acted as Superior and administrator for 15 years. In 1935, Sister Marie was honoured with the Silver Jubilee Medal by King George V and Queen Mary. Two years later, she supervised the building of a new wing at the hospital.

But the new wing was something the Religious Hospitallers of St. Joseph had dreamed of making long before it was finally approved. Sister Marie wrote to Bishop Fallon in 1925 informing him that at the chapter meeting of the sisters it was unanimously agreed to seek permission to pursue a building project that would enlarge the hospital. Fallon hastily replied on August 29, 1925:

"I am unable at the present time to give my approval to this resolution; my reason for such refusal lies in the fact that the members of your community are even now too few for the work they have in hand. If the enlargement of your building took place it would mean that the hospital would be less than ever under religious control as the number of secular nurses would have to be largely increased. Such would tend to gradually destroy the idea of a Sisters' hospital."

Fallon feared losing "religious" control over the hospital. He wasn't about to budge on this, despite Windsor Mayor Frank J. Mitchell publicly stating that Hôtel-Dieu had been "strained to the uttermost to accommodate the patients applying for admission to the well equipped and splendidly conducted institution." The mayor urged Fallon to grant approval, arguing that there was "no doubt that much greater accommodation must be provided." Mitchell also applauded the sisters at Hôtel-Dieu for "valuable work" in the city.

Sister Marie also found support for her initiative for an addition at Hôtel-Dieu from doctors in the community who signed a petition that was handed to the bishop. Fallon's reply of January 12, 1927 hinted that the doctors— if they really wanted this—needed to assume the financial risks. The bishop also argued that the future demanded a building much larger, and that the present site was "inappropriate," and surely would become more so in the future when a larger more "general hospital" was needed. Fallon also said Hôtel-Dieu was too close to a growing business section of Windsor itself.

The new hospital addition would have to wait until the 1930s when Sister Marie, who

had stepped aside for a new Superior, returned to running the hospital and guiding it through the Great Depression. The new wing opened in 1938.

The battles with Fallon plagued Sister Marie. Even from the beginning, just two days before she was elected Superior, Fallon wrote a letter to the community (September 1, 1923) that he was worried over the health of the religious order here. He claimed that he had remained "aloof—more even than perhaps (my) obligations required," but felt that the religious order was declining rapidly, and that there had been "practically no new vocations."

Even Sister Marie's election was marred by the interference of Fallon, which had been presided over by Dean Downey, the pastor of St. Alphonsus Church. He counted the votes, and the congregation had clearly made their choice. Fallon, hearing of this, notified the Windsor sisters that he didn't approve, and demanded that Mother Marie tender her resignation. The sisters in their annals said the bishop's response was "by way of intimidation." The same day, a young professed member of the community— Therese de L'Enfant-Jesus—was in a retreat preparing for her final vows. Fallon put a quick stop to this on the eve of that ceremony. The sisters were livid, and wrote to Monsignor Di Maria, the apostolic delegate to the Holy See. This letter of Sept. 18, 1923 reads:

"We take the respectful liberty, your

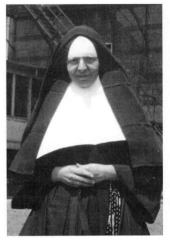

Sister Marie de la Ferre (Laura LeBoeuf)

Series of Questions to which an Answer is requested by

J. M. F. Fallon, Bp London

December 10th, 1926.

* *

1. How many applicants for admission as postulants in the Hotel Dieu Hospital, Windsor, have been refused during the past three years? *2,*

2. What are their names?

Mrs Piché
Miss Monica Mooney

3. What reason was given for their rejection? *Their age, and unfitness to be trained for our work, in our Community*

4. To whom did they apply? *Myself.* *Both were nervous wreck*

Sister Marie de la Ferre,

December ....1926.

Sister Marie de la Ferre's response to a query from the bishop about the rejection of applicants to the hospital. At the end she provides a dour comment that the postulants were both "nervous wrecks."

Excellency, to protest against this unjust and not motivated by interference. We want to be good religious. We wish to do the work entrusted to us by our founders. It is our desire to live in peace and under obedience to our ecclesiastical superiors. All we ask is their support and protection to accomplish our duties… This support has been refused us for a number of years and it is due to it (that) if our novitiate has not increased in a more satisfactory manner. Our community is reduced to a very small number…"

Sister Marie's elevation to Superior was eventually approved by the bishop. She knew that the number one item on her list was finding a way to keep him from interfering and more importantly, of preventing him from dissolving the religious order's work in Windsor. The sisters lived in trepidation of the future. They struggled to find new recruits, but many of the young French-Canadian women who had considered entering the religious life were going elsewhere. The word was out—their Irish bishop was disapproving of them. Or so it seemed.

As for Fallon's refusal to grant permission to Therese de L'Enfant-Jesus, the nuns managed to circumvent this by putting her on a train and sending her to its Montreal congregation where she would not be subject to Fallon's decree.

Meanwhile, the London bishop continued

to criticize the Religious Hospitallers of Windsor for their lack of enterprise in drawing new postulants to the community. In December 1926, he condescendingly dispatched what he termed "a series of questions" to Sister Marie regarding new applicants. The first question asked how many they had refused. The reply was two. The second question asked their names, and the third, the reasons given for rejecting them. Sister Marie wrote: "Both were nervous wrecks." Fallon hesitated until January 12, 1927 to respond, reproaching the sisters of refusing English-speaking postulants. He then informed Sister Marie that he had the names of seven others, "all English-speaking, who in one way or another have been debarred from entering your community."

Sister Marie envisioned the future of the order, and what was needed to meet the demands of a growing community among the Border Cities. Thus, she organized the first advisory board for the hospital. In 1951, however, the sister departed Hôtel-Dieu for Whitelaw, Alberta to work in a hospital for the chronically ill. She remained only a couple of years, and returned to Hôtel-Dieu. In 1958, Sister Marie was sent to Villa Maria to devote her energies to the elderly. Six years later, she returned to the hospital to do pastoral work. In 1968, she celebrated her Diamond Jubilee and was named Citizen of the Year by the city. In 1975, Sister Marie passed away in the hospital where she had cared for the sick. Her nephew, Rev. Mar-

Bishop's House
90 Central Avenue
London, Ontario, Canada

January 12th, 1927.

Rev. Sr. Marie de la Ferre,
Hotel Dieu Hospital,
Windsor, Ont.

Dear Rev. Sister,

I am in receipt of your answers under date of December 14th, 1926, to my questions of December 10th, 1926. Upon your answers I make the following comments:

1. Within the past few months Very Rev. F. X. Laurendeau, Dean of Essex, has informed me that your community will not receive English-speaking postulants.

2. Besides the two names that you furnished me I have a list of 7 others, all English-speaking, who in one way or another have been debarred from entering your community. This condition is one that could scarcely be expected to meet the approval of any religious superior.

With all good wishes, I remain

Yours faithfully in Christ,

M. F. Fallon,
Bishop of London.

P. S. This letter was dictated on the 8th inst. but owing to the absence of the secretary could not be sent until this date.

ARCHIVES
R.H.S.J.
WINDSOR, ONT.

01.03.004 BOX4, FILE4

Bishop Fallon's tense response to a query about Hôtel Dieu not accepting English-speaking postulants

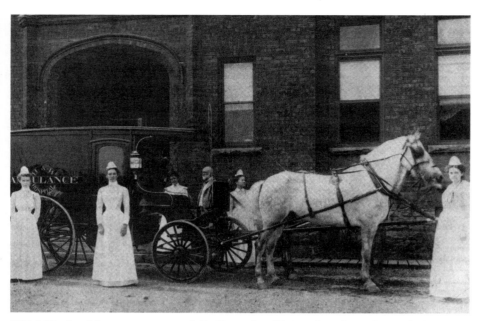
Hôtel-Dieu's white ambulance was painted black after going in for repairs

cel LeBoeuf, officiated at her funeral that was held in Hôtel-Dieu's chapel.

Many Firsts

The Ambulance

The first ambulance to be used in Windsor was introduced by Hôtel-Dieu in 1891. The hospital bought it at a cost of $450. Friends donated the money for this horse-drawn carriage that was white with the name "Hotel-Dieu... City" painted in black. Up until that moment, the hospital had to use one borrowed from St. Mary's Hospital in Detroit for emergency cases. It had to be driven onto the ferry boat, and taken across the Detroit River. Not the best way of getting to urgent cases.

There was no question that Windsor needed the ambulance, and the hospital had to raise the money through "subscriptions" or donations. The hospital already had $250 in its bank account, but the remainder had to be found over the next few months. It was through the fundraising of the Ladies Auxiliary that Hôtel-Dieu was able to raise the balance. "For us, as well as the city, it was a distinct advantage which exempted the City from borrowing that of St. Mary's Hospital in Detroit for urgent cases."

The sisters in describing the new ambulance in the *Annals* wrote: "This ambulance was painted white and was very beautiful. However, it required a lot of upkeep in order to keep it clean."

The new carriage was entrusted to Gordon McGregor, who was working with his father at Walkerville Wagon Works and who would go on to found Ford Motor Company of Canada. McGregor benefited from the ambulance. According to the nuns, each time it was used, he received payment. Just three years later, however, Hôtel-Dieu found itself again without an ambulance because it had to go in for repairs. The work was done but "this time it was painted black," according to the Annalists. The name was also erased in the process. A Mr. Ferriss was put in charge of taking care of it. Unfortunately, so says the nun's report of 1899: "His (Ferriss') buildings were burned down and the dear ambulance was consumed with the other items. It was not insured."

Hôtel-Dieu's doctors finally appealed to the city's municipal council, as well as to politicians in both Walkerville and Sandwich to replace it. It took until December 1903 to get approval, and the work was tendered out for one to be built. It would cost $800.

First Surgery

The first surgery to be done at Hôtel-Dieu was conducted by Dr. Raymond Casgrain. He removed an ovarian cyst, and it was entirely successful.

Before the hospital conducted surgeries, all that could be done was make the patient comfortable. Sister Marie de la Ferre told *The Windsor Star* on the occasion of her 50th anniversary as a nun that operations, except for amputations, were virtually unknown when she started her nursing training in 1908. She said, "We treated illnesses as best we could. If a patient was admitted with appendicitis we applied ice to try and help him. That's all we could do. If he died—he died."

Basins, Hot Water, and Kleptomaniacs

Something as simple as basins for the doctors was a concern in the winter and spring of 1908. The doctors complained there wasn't a place for them to wash up before or after surgeries, or at least a place that was convenient. Again it was a matter of dollars.

The new dressing room for the doctors was being built and, naturally, the thought was that the doctors might also have a set of basins installed. The nuns balked at this—it was not in their budget. Their thought was that both the doctors and the nurses could "scrub" up at the same basins, and maybe the physicians did not require more privacy. Sister LaDauversiere, however, in responding to a letter from the secretary of the Medical Staff committee, pointed out that the unwillingness on the part of the sisters was due mostly because the doctors had decided they wouldn't contribute to the costs involved. The secretary responded a few days later that they would. Sister LaDauversiere informed the medical staff that it would cost $75 each for these three basins. The sinks would come equipped with foot pedals. In 1919, the medical doctors at Hôtel-Dieu complained, too, that they did not have suitable places to hang their coats. At that point in time, they would use the cloakroom that was used by the general public. It seems some enterprising thieves were at work to cause this letter to be written November 24, 1919 by E. H McGavin, secretary of the Medical Staff. He stated that the consensus among management at Hôtel-Dieu was that "more suitable and safe quarters for the doctors' coats and hats" be provided. He noted that the cloakroom was "most inviting to those who may be afflicted by kleptomania."

The other complaint from doctors—this one lodged with the Mother Superior in a letter dated January 28, 1920—was for "hot water" in

"Some people would go to bed healthy and never wake up."

the operating room sinks, but also some improvement to the heating system. Apparently, the doctors were reaching for sweaters and lab coats to keep warm during surgeries.

Bells

In the fall of 1910, the sisters received a letter from Dr. E. Prouse from the Medical Staff board complaining of the liturgical noises emanating from the convent. It seems the ringing of bells and other religious service sounds had become disturbing annoyances to the patients, doctors and nurses. Prouse, in his Oct. 12, 1910 note to the Mother Superior wrote:

"The staff requested me to write to you asking if some means could not be adopted whereby the noise from the bells and other noises could not be lessened. The reason for making the suggestion is that many patients suffer from a nervous condition, which is increased by a sudden striking of a bell. They thought some other apparatus could be used which would eliminate much of the sounds."

Who's in Charge?

The sisters at Hôtel-Dieu certainly knew their "place" when it came to London's Bishop Fallon, and how to respond, and defer to him. The doctors and the medical staff simply went about their work. Their contact—in terms of upper management—was always with the Mother Superior and her assistants. If they wanted something changed, they went to the sisters. In 1922, it seems Fallon was a little put off with the way in which decisions were being made without his personal approval. He placed the blame entirely upon the sisters, specifically Sister St. Joseph, the Superior. Seeing how this upset her, the medical staff's secretary immediately sent Sister St. Joseph a note promising to rectify "the misunderstanding" and dispatched another note on January 23, 1922 to Fallon explaining how the staff ought to have included him with their concerns.

Deadly Diseases

The 1918 Spanish Influenza Outbreak

Between 30,000 and 50,000 Canadians died the winter of 1918—not in the fields of France where the Kaiser's armies were in full retreat, but in their urban homes, or farmhouses, or hospitals all across this country. The "Spanish Flu," as it was called, started right after Labour Day, and killed nine American soldiers stationed in Quebec City. That same day, 400 students in a school in Quebec became ill. By the beginning of October, the disease had spread far and wide. Worst hit was Brantford where medical authorities reported some 2,500 incidents. In his article, "The 1918 Influenza Outbreak: The Spanish Flu Panics Canada" health historian George Siamandas writes how "tens of thou-

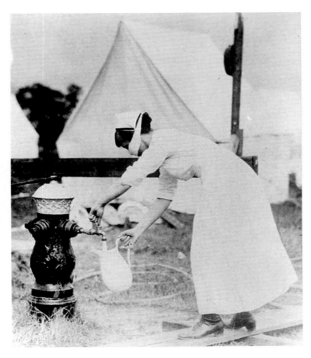

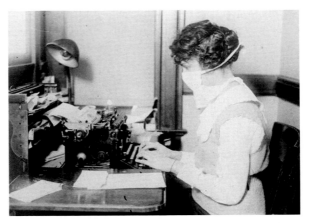

sands fell ill…(And) as the death toll mounted, communities started to ban public gatherings, (and) schools, colleges, and universities were closed." At some stores, like the Hudson's Bay Company, and the Canadian Imperial Bank of Commerce, Siamandas said, employees wore masks. He also pointed out that trains were prohibited from letting passengers get off in communities unless they promised "to stay put for the duration of the epidemic." Other towns enforced a quarantine. World wide, a reported 21 million died—more than the number who died during the course of the First World War. It has been said the disease was spread by soldiers returning home from the war. As Dan Bjarnason and Robin Rowland wrote in their article for CBC, the disease was "a serial killer." They said: "Medical facilities were swamped. The killer flu struck quickly and inexplicably. Some people would go to bed healthy and never wake up."

At first, it seemed Windsor was spared in the spread of that disease. So it appeared from reading *The Border Cities Star,* or listening to the city's mayor, Charles R. Tuson. Early on, the paper boldly reported there were no incidents. That was for good reason—the city, unlike other communities in the country, was prepared for it. As one writer said in reviewing Steven Palmer and Steve Malone's *Border City Medicine: Windsor's History of Innovative Health Practice,* "the facilities and practitioners were in place to address the challenges to public health."

But when the influenza struck the city during the fall of 1918, it came with a vengeance; Hôtel-Dieu reeled from the onslaught. One-hundred-and-twenty-six people died of the disease in two months. Detroit was worse. The flu claimed 3,814 lives. As the reviewer of Palmer and Malone's book states, "Newspapers published long lists of the dead, quarantine signs became common, death wreaths and black bunting draped many homes. Funerals were hurried affairs with few mourners. Coffins stored near funeral homes were often stolen by impatient and fearful family members, while bodies were placed on porches for daily pickup."

The one-term Mayor Tuson attempted to play down the local flu epidemic at the beginning of October 1918, saying "all precautions" were in place to ward off its foothold in Windsor after the warnings issued by Col. J.W.S. McCullough, chief officer of the Ontario Board of Health. The provincial body lamented the shortage of doctors and nurses to stem the tide of the disease, and cautioned that there weren't enough hospital beds to meet the rising numbers. Deaths were already mounting up in Montreal; Ontario was now vulnerable. Regions all over Ontario, in fact, were issuing major quarantines.

Tuson's strategy was aimed at calming the population. Windsor's Dr. G. F. Cruickshanks of Sandwich, then acting medical officer of health until Dr. Fred Adams took over in September 1919, wasn't about to wait. Children queued up outside city hall on a Saturday to be vaccinated. Cruickshanks advised school authorities to refuse any students unless they could prove

"The killer flu struck quickly and inexplicably."

they had received their proper shots. Meanwhile, Walkerville swiftly remodeled Mayor C. W. Hoare's residence at Devonshire Road and Wyandotte to be the area's first emergency hospital. By mid-October, the Border Cities (Sandwich, Windsor, Walkerville and Ford City) were under siege, and Hôtel-Dieu was handling 32 cases of the Spanish Flu. Three of its patients included two doctors and the wife of one of those physicians. Cruickshanks expected many more cases of the influenza, and maintained that families were telephoning to say their loved ones were crippled by the disease, but were remaining at home instead of driving to the hospital. The medical officer of health also warned against sending children to school if there was sickness in the home. He said that people suffering from the flu would be "isolated," but he promised not to placard their homes. Cruickshanks also urged those stricken with the flu to see doctors immediately.

Sister Cecile Leboeuf, now 93, and former Superior of the order and chief administrator of Hôtel-Dieu, said the hospital was under an enormous strain during those autumn months. But help came from all quarters of the city. She said, "Baum and Brody supplied beds from its furniture store. They were lined up in the corridors. No one was refused help." But that's not entirely true. By the end of October 1918, Hôtel-Dieu was so overrun that it actually turned away people at its front doors. *The Border Cities Star* ran the headline: *'FLU'*

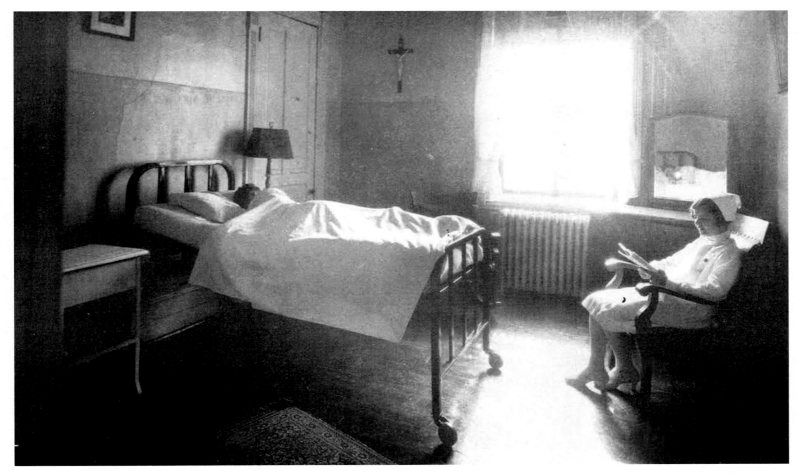

PATIENTS CROWD HOSPITAL; NO BEDS LEFT.

The city swiftly reacted with converting the Great War Veteran's Home into an emergency influenza hospital. Hôtel-Dieu at this point housed nearly 100 patients. Nine were accommodated in a 15-foot-square room, while other rooms had three times their ordinary numbers. The Veteran's home was capable of accommodating at least 20 patients, and a nurse from Hôtel-Dieu was sent over to staff the alternate facility. Volunteers soon joined her.

"We had a lot of volunteers," said Sister LeBoeuf. These included the Holy Names Sisters and the Ursulines, but the Knights of Columbus also came to the rescue. "Many of these people came to work in the kitchen or the laundry on a 'night watch' with the sick," she said.

By October 1918, Hôtel Dieu had been overrun by Spanish Flu victims to the point that Hôtel Dieu had to refuse patients at the door. The disease claimed the lives of 126 in two months in Windsor.

Sister LeBoeuf said the Hôtel-Dieu sisters who worked among the sick somehow managed to stay healthy throughout the ordeal. The same could not be said of other volunteers. *The Border Cities Star* indicated that four of 16 women who offered to help at the hospital came down with the illness.

It wasn't long before the Salvation Army opened up its own hospital (Grace). Its officials were promising it was readying itself to deal with the illness. Finally, Tuson acted, placing a ban on schools, churches, dance halls and places where more than 25 people were gathered. Meanwhile, his own daughter fell ill with the flu. Tuson told the newspaper that precautions were being put into place now rather than waiting for "the plague becoming even more general." The community, however, wasn't in favour of this decision, and soon demanded that it be lifted in order to accommodate a rally aimed at raising money for a Victory Loan drive. With the war in Europe still raging, fundraisers were pressuring the mayor to lift the ban, if only for a few days. Gordon M. McGregor, one of the founders of Ford Motor Company of Canada, and a staunch proponent of stricter health measures, surprisingly favoured lifting the injunction. Ironically, the same day that Tuson agreed to rescind the prohibition, 63 new cases of the flu were reported by the Walkerville Board of Health.

During this time, the Catholic Church announced it would honour the sanction against assembly, thereby permitting its following to abstain from Sunday mass. Funeral mourners were also warned to stay away—the remains of the deceased never went past the church doors. This was all done so as to avoid contagion. Throughout the epidemic, there were daily notices in *The Border Cities Star*, tabulating the death numbers, but also reporting the arrival of more serum.

By November 1918, Windsor's mayor came down with the flu. He was ordered to bed for three or four days by his family doctor who said he had "a mild case." Apparently he fainted three times during the night. The next day, the board of health reported 49 new cases, but also the death of a 48-year-old woman from Leamington. Earlier in the week, a 16-year-old woman, married only six months, died from the flu.

The only good news in all that tragedy was November 9, 1918 when the German Kaiser abdicated, and the war in Europe came to an end. Full-page ads in the newspaper that day declared: "The War Is Won!" It was clear, however, that the war against the Spanish Flu was still raging on the home front. The J. Gelber Furniture Company may not have appreciated the irony when it ran an advertisement in November 11, 1918 that the war was over and that the population should "Prepare for the Home-Coming." Indeed, the soldiers were returning home to confounding illness. Some, who had miraculously survived the bloodiest of battles in France, were dead within a few weeks upon their return.

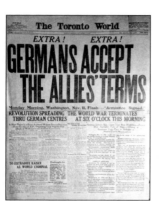

Good news in the headlines at last: the abdication of the German Kaiser ended the war in Europe.

The night that the war ended in Europe was the cause of celebration in Windsor's streets, but nurses at Hôtel-Dieu stuffed cotton batting into the ears of the sick in hopes they would not be disturbed.

Christopher Rutty and Sue C. Sullivan in in their book, *This Is Public Health: A Canadian History*, said by the time the pandemic leveled off, "at least one-sixth of the population, predominantly young adults, had been stricken." These writers go on to explain that the disease itself wasn't really understood and isolated until 1933.

Smallpox Epidemic

There seemed to be no cause for worry on February 2, 1924 when Gordon Deneau—complaining of a headache, sore throat and rotting gums—was examined by his doctor and promptly sent home. That was a Saturday night. Deneau was counseled that he likely needed to have his teeth removed entirely because acute pyorrhea had set in. Three days later, he was admitted to the hospital; his body had erupted in major blotches that were described as being "from a bean to an egg in size" by Fred Adams, the local medical officer of health for the Essex Border Municipalities. The man's headache persisted. So did the sore throat, and his temperature had risen to 101. Otherwise, he feigned being normal, even rising out of bed to joke with the nurses. The prognosis? Little concern. By Monday, February 11, however, the

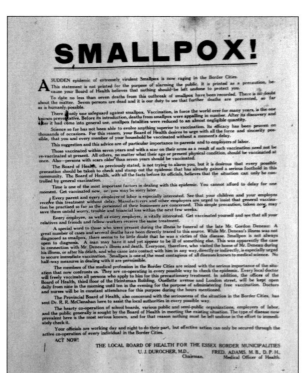

The Board of Health distributed flyers urging parents to have their children vaccinated against smallpox.

man, whom Adams referred to simply as G.D., (but in fact, according to *The Border Cities Star* was Gordon Deneau) suddenly took a turn for the worse, and passed away. That's when physicians determined it was smallpox.

What they didn't know was this would be only the beginning. Suddenly there were 66 more cases of it in the city, 32 of whom died. It was one of the worst epidemics of smallpox to occur in Canada in modern times. It may not have rivaled the occurrences in the 18th century in Canada when the French general Montcalm reported some 2,500 cases in Quebec City. Twenty per cent of these perished. The Brit-

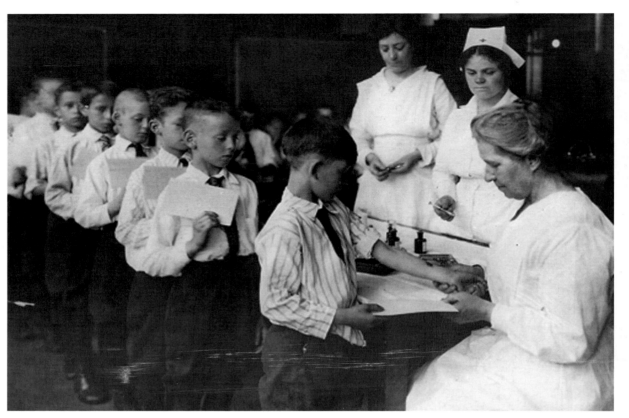

Children line up to be vaccinated against smallpox, one of the worst epidemics to occur in Canada. By 1925, some 50,000 people in Windsor and surrounding areas were vaccinated.

ish to this day still carry the terrible reputation of spreading it deliberately, when in 1763, they used blankets exposed to smallpox to quash the Indian uprising led by Pontiac, an incident regarded as the first known use of "germ warfare." By 1798, however, a smallpox cure had been discovered by Rev. John Clinch. He was a classmate of Edward Jenner, the first to prove that vaccination could prevent smallpox. Thus, by the 1920s, there was really no excuse for smallpox occurrences—vaccination was widely available. In all of the deaths in Windsor not one of

these individuals had ever been vaccinated.

The next victim had recently visited Deneau. Of course, he never realized his friend had smallpox. On February 20, the man took ill, complaining of a sore back and severe headache. He was at the hospital that Wednesday night, and by Friday, February 22, his body was covered in lobster-red blotches. Again doctors misdiagnosed it, thinking it was a form of "erythema" or sometimes classified as "scaratiniform." Twenty-four hours later, the man passed away. At one point, Hôtel-Dieu's attending physicians did ask if he had been in contact with anyone who had smallpox, and he denied that he had. Later, it was learned he had, in fact, seen his old friend, who had died only days before, but of course never realized it was the same disease that he would die from.

An 80-year-old man, who lived in the same house as the first victim, also came down with the disease, but promptly recovered. He had been vaccinated 60 years before. Even more surprising, Deneau's 12-year-old daughter survived, having never developed "one single day's illness herself." That's because six years before, she had been vaccinated at school. The scar of that vaccination on her arm, Adams said, was "the size of an old fashioned Canadian five cent piece."

On the other hand, 21 close relatives of this little girl—all unvaccinated, Adams pointed out—were dead from smallpox. It has been suggested, according to a website blogger related to the Deneau family, that many of those who came down with the disease were "close relatives" who had been to his funeral.

On February 24, 1924, a trained nurse, 34 years old, called "M.B." by Adams in his report, checked into the hospital, and had her appendix removed. While recovering, she broke out with a "mixed kind of rash…Her face was flushed as with scarlet fever and her eyes were inflamed. There was a rash on the body which resembled measles. She had come off a scarlet fever case two weeks before but believed that she had had scarlet fever as a child." According to Adams,

M.B. showed no signs of sore throat and "no strawberry tongue." All indications were that she had measles. She informed the doctors she had never had smallpox, nor had she been vaccinated. Adams wrote in his report: "The case was not believed to be smallpox, but in view of the uncertainty of the diagnosis (she) was isolated and the nurse who was caring for her was vaccinated at once…Thursday it was learned that the patient's brother had smallpox and the home was quarantined." The patient finally was permitted to return home; that's where she died a few days later.

Another victim was Joseph Laurin, a Windsor barber, who died after eight days with the illness, and apparently contracted it from having shaved a smallpox patient at his barber shop. Like the others, he came down with a fever, sore throat, and sores along his limbs.

A family of 10 people, named simply as "M" by Adams, was exposed to the disease. Nine had been vaccinated successfully and never fell ill. The tenth, who had never been vaccinated, died within four days of the appearance of that "lobster rash type of smallpox." In another case, a 58-year-old woman, who had lived in the Hôtel-Dieu convent for three years and had been vaccinated, managed to push off the disease when it struck.

What occurred in Windsor should not come as a surprise since, across the river—and there was constant commerce between the two cities—there were 710 cases of smallpox between

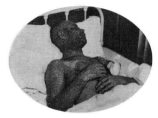

Joseph Laurin, a Windsor barber, died of smallpox.

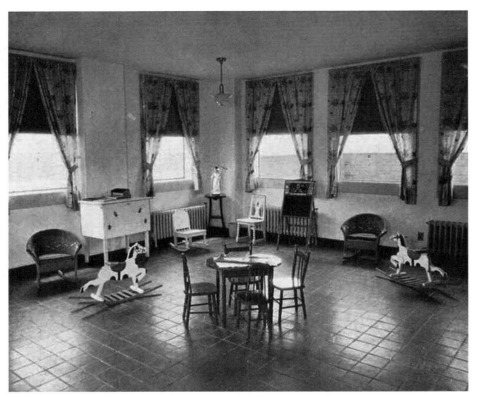

The children's ward opened on May 12, 1927.

There is no conclusive information as to why more people weren't vaccinated to begin with, but as soon as news hit the streets in Windsor that an epidemic was in full bloom, the population responded swiftly. In two weeks alone during the winter of 1924, according to an article by C. C. Pierce published in *The Boston Medical and Surgical Journal* in April 1925, 50,000 were vaccinated, and the epidemic subsided. The cost to Windsor residents was a mere four cents per vaccination. The treatment of those afflicted with smallpox, and subsequent deaths cost city taxpayers more than $35,000 in 1924.

On February 23, 1924, the Board of Health in Windsor finally met to deal with the presence of this killer disease. "By that time," said Adams, "we knew we were dealing with smallpox…that it was an exceedingly virulent and irregular form…" It was decided that widespread vaccination was necessary. To that end, three nurses on Saturday got on the telephone and dialed up every doctor in the Border Cities, asking them if they would consent to vaccinating any person "free of charge, with the definite understanding that the Board of Health would supply vaccine and pay for vaccinations at the rate of 25 cents apiece." Within a half hour, three quarters of the physicians telephoned their consent to the procedure. Further calls were made Sunday morning in an effort to reach the other doctors. Monday morning the Chamber of Commerce telephoned all major manufacturing outlets in the area urging them to notify employees. The

September 1, 1923 and March 15, 1924. But from March to June 1924, there were another 795 cases, with 105 deaths. There is nothing conclusive to suggest that it spread from Detroit. Eventually, the border between Windsor and Detroit was shut down to anyone who couldn't prove vaccination. All that was necessary was to roll up a sleeve, and display the scar on your arm. This action was taken by Henry F. Vaughn, Detroit's Health Commissioner, who dispatched nurses to the border to meet passengers coming off the ferry boat. Those without proof of vaccination were turned back immediately.

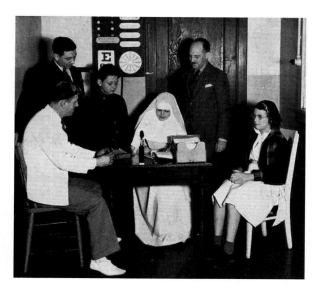

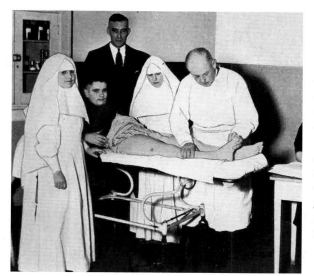

Left: Windsor Lions Cub has supported preventing blindness and restoring sight among Windsor children since 1929.

Right: The Windsor Rotary Club supported the Orthopaedic Clinic, making it possible to return children's broken and deformed limbs to normal.

response was overwhelming. Seventy doctors in the Border Cities set up gratis vaccination stations, and people were lining up at doctors' offices from morning to night. Adams maintained that there was "nothing compulsory" about the approach: "We simply took the public into our confidence, told them the situation as it really was…"

Mobilized to fight the disease, said Adams, was an army of nurses to look after the sick, orderlies, ambulance drivers, clergymen, and volunteers. Measures were taken, of course, to ensure that each one of these individuals was properly vaccinated.

As one might expect, there was mild resistance to it from the anti-vaccination movement, said Adams. Fortunately, their voices were muted during this difficult time. They stood out of the way of what has come to be

called "The Speckled Monster." There was too much at stake.

The efforts of Adams, who was working around the clock, to stem the tide of this disease, seemed to work. He ordered all pupils and school staff to be vaccinated. Students, as a matter of fact, were turned away at the school's front doors if they could not show the telltale scar of the vaccination.

Adams knew, too, he had to deal with the steady flow of sick. Hôtel-Dieu was stretched to the limits, and Grace soon came under quarantine. This is what led to authorities turning the Grand Central Hotel into an "isolation hospital." Those quarantined there included Deneau's wife and a few of his relatives.

The city campaign to vaccinate the population was advertised widely in the newspaper, including a full-page ad urging "every parent

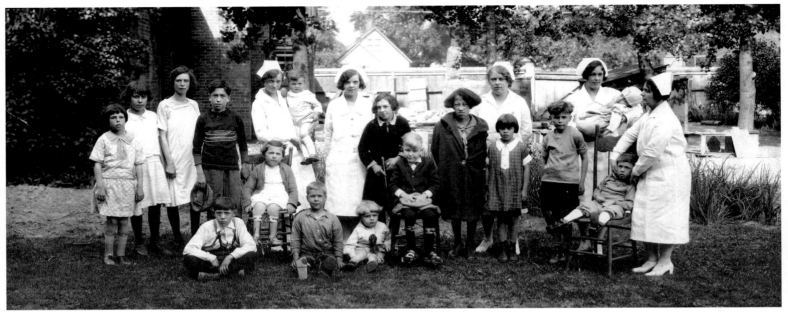

Hôtel-Dieu's Crippled Children's Clinic, 1915

and every employer" in the city to be vaccinated at once. The Board of Health also set up its headquarters in Heintzman Building, this downtown piano business edifice, then located at the southeast corner of what is now University Avenue and Ouellette (on the site of the present day *Windsor Star)*. Soon the lines began to extend down Ouellette Avenue as people showed up at the building on a Sunday morning. The offices, situated on the third floor of that downtown building, were kept open from 9 a.m. until 10 p.m., and staffed with local doctors and nurses. Windsor area doctors had been drafted into action, and promised compensation for their time.

The *Border Cities Star* announcement made reference to Deneau, the first victim of small-pox, and warned friends and family to stay clear of the house where he lived. The ad read: "Everyone…who visited the home of Mr. Deneau during his illness, or after his death, and who came into contact with him in any way…is especially urged to secure immediate vaccination. Smallpox is one of the most contagious of all diseases known to medical science."

Meanwhile further announcements went out that Sunday morning to parishioners everywhere to be vaccinated at once. Adams was even alerting mourners to stay away from funerals. For example, a friend of Gordon Deneau—Henry Dubey of Detroit—had crossed the border to bring his condolences, and came down with smallpox, and died here in Windsor.

PART III

Depression, the War and Post-War

1930s-1950s

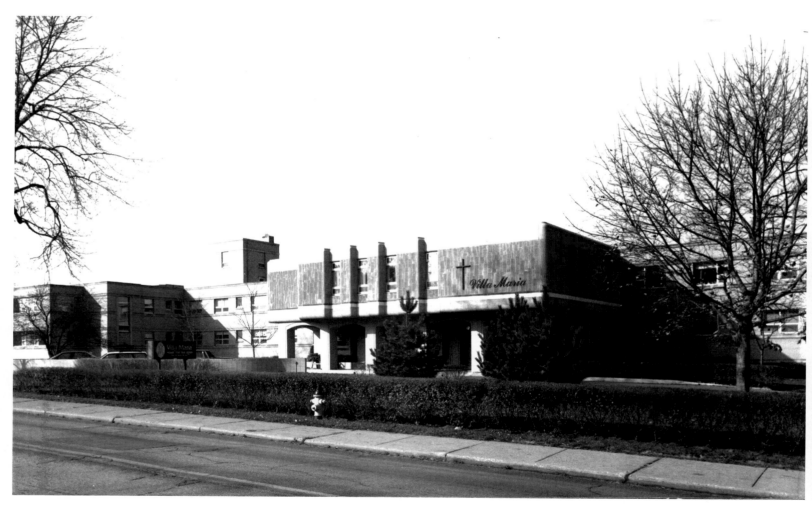

Villa Maria, named for former Sister Superior Maria Guevin, opened August 5, 1956 and began accepting its first residents.

Villa Maria

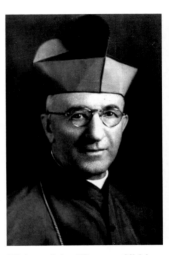

Bishop John Thomas Kidd of London, ON, circa 1931

IT TOOK NEARLY A DECADE OF PRESSURE FROM SENIOR CITIZENS AND PASTORS FROM ALL OVER WINDsor and Essex County for the establishment of a Catholic home for the aged. The idea was raised as early as 1933, but the Depression was in full bloom and money was in short supply. Still, the pressure was on to help the aged, and that responsibility seemed to fall on the shoulders of the sisters at Hôtel-Dieu Hospital.

The community had to wait nearly 10 years. That's when two close supporters of the sisters—Monsignor Charles A. Parent and Rev. Gregory L. Blondé—learned of a house that could be picked up for tax arrears near the Ambassador Bridge, a stone's throw from Assumption College. They thought that Sister Claire Maître, then Superior and administrator of Hôtel-Dieu, should snatch it up without delay. The Mother Superior agreed, but first had to convene a meeting of her counsel and the hospital advisory board. Plans were then put in place to purchase this white brick house that sat alongside the Detroit River. Arrangements were then made for Bishop Kidd to bless the building—now called St. John the Evangelist Home for the Aged—on January 15, 1944. The following day the Bishop celebrated mass in a makeshift chapel. Seventy two Knights of Columbus members were there for this inaugural event.

The doors were opened for residents on that same day. It didn't take long for St. John the Evangelist to be filled with elderly residents. It became clear that expansion was needed, or another house should be bought. That led the Hôtel-Dieu sisters to purchase a neighboring home, and it too was soon filled to capacity. By 1955, St. John the Evangelist had grown to four houses. The sisters sensed that a single facility that could house more than 100 residents was inevitable, but kept from proceeding with it to keep costs down. That's when they sought the advice of Sir Harry Gignac and W. H. Cantelon, both of whom served on the home's board. The two influential commu-

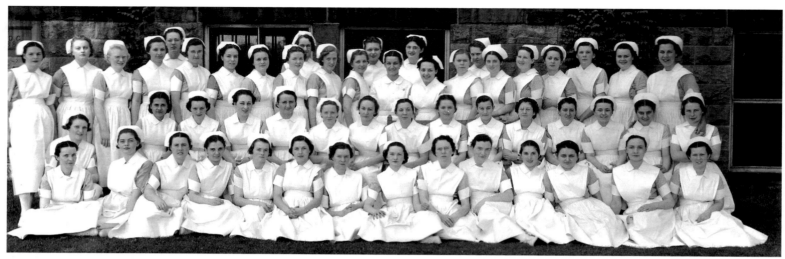

Hôtel-Dieu's New Nursing Students, circa 1938

nity personalities put out the word quickly and managed to convince municipal officials and the general public that such a move was vital. This led to construction of a new home on the same site as the original St. John the Evangelist. It was renamed Villa Maria, named for former Sister Superior Maria Guevin. The new facility opened August 5, 1956 and began accepting its first residents. Sister Blanche Garceau was appointed Superior. Until 1971, the Superior also acted as administrator. This changed in 1972 when lay people were hired to manage the old age home. Villa Maria closed in 2003 as part of the alliance merger. The building is now in the hands of the University of Windsor and serves as a student residence.

The 1946 Tornado

The city was already reeling from a storm that had bullied its way through the farm coun-try around Windsor, knocking tree limbs to the city streets. This was more of an annoyance than anything else. Certainly not quite what was to follow on June 17, 1946 when a 10-minute fury befell Windsor. Ten minutes, and it was over. Homes, garages, cars, buses—and the dead—lay all around. Seventeen killed in the 1946 Tornado. Hundreds hurt. And a night of darkness. No power. No lights. Nothing but emergency lights, candles, bonfires, lanterns.

The black twister that ripped its way through the western edges of the city from Ojibway and Sandwich spun and swooped in an arch around the southern outskirts and then suddenly vanished. As Stu Beitler and others have written in stories of this tornado, this black funnel was "a pure freak in these northern temperate latitudes," a "dark devil" when it slammed its way through this city, rendering Windsor at a standstill. Firefighters from all over the region along with police, doctors, nurses, Red Cross workers and hundreds of volunteers searched through the rubble all night to find their loved ones, and to pull the injured to safety. Emergency lights burned until early morning the next day, and drinking water had to be drawn directly from the Detroit River and purified through emergency chlorination because the filtration plant had been shut down.

This 250-mph black ghost swallowed up nearly everything in its 100-yard swath when it struck at suppertime that June day. Some attempted to race down to their cellars to save themselves, but were caught in those precious seconds on the basement stairs as their homes were uprooted and wrenched from the foundations. Some woke up in yards next door while others perished. Witnesses said that when the tornado bounced from River Rouge to the Detroit River, it created four huge waterspouts before veering its terrifying way through Windsor. Miraculously it missed three Cleveland bound steamship lines. Another witness spotted a cow doing summersaults in the air before being thrown back to the field where she had been grazing, and she merely shook herself, and carried right on.

Beitler quotes Charles J. Ellison, a Windsor funeral director, as saying that he found the body of one man who had been blown two blocks from his home—the man's three-year-old daughter lay dead beside him. In another case, a seven-year-old boy had the clothes from his body ripped right off, and he ambled about aimlessly after the storm searching for his mother. Meanwhile, another man told his tale of seeing a boy catapulted from his bicycle into the air as the tornado hit, and the smashed bicycle was found but the body of the boy was not.

W. H. Coyle, told *The Star* that the tornado seemed to have "electricity in the centre of it … It wasn't black…It was grey, the shape of a cone, with the tip toward the earth. It seemed to bounce along and every time the tip of the cone touched the earth, there was a trail of smoke. It just seemed to pick or suck a house up and grind it to bits, dropping pieces of wood and debris all over the country."

Coyle found the body of a little girl, maybe nine years old, in the underbrush. He said, "The clothes were blown completely off her, and her face was in the mud. She had been blown 150 to 200 feet from the home and we found her about 75 feet from her parents…The bodies appeared as those of mummies with the features depressed instead of bloated, and the skin had taken of a sickly purplish blue."

When it was all done, it was like a bomb had hit the area. The only thing left of some houses was the foundations. Trees were uprooted. Cars were found blocks from where they had been parked. The June 17, 1946 tornado is still considered the strongest and deadliest tornado to touch down in Windsor.

That night, both Hôtel-Dieu and Grace Hospitals were working non-stop. The corri-

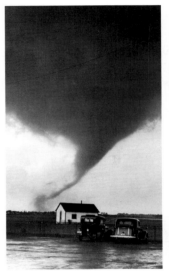

Tornado touching down along Walker Road, June 17, 1946. (Courtesy of The Windsor Star)

dors were jammed with beds, nurses, orderlies and doctors rushed about, all in the dim light of this black day. The power was out. As the *Windsor Daily Star* reported, "For nearly an hour after the tragedy occurred, attendants at the hospital were forced to carry on their work by candlelight." Police, firemen and ordinary citizens showed up with flashlights and lanterns. Storage batteries for an emergency lighting system in the operating rooms were set up by Horseshoe Battery, a Windsor company. Market Hardware, another store, dropped off dozens of gasoline lamps to relieve the situation.

"...attendants were forced to carry on their work by candlelight..."

The first patients among the throng of injured were Mrs. Fred Pageau and her two-year-old daughter, Jacqueline and five-month-old son, Gerald. The mother had suffered a bruised shoulder. She told *The Star* it was only her prayers that saved her family when their wood-frame house exploded and collapsed from the twister's ferocity. She found the baby under a wall, and her daughter wandering among the debris. She picked them up and rushed outside. Someone driving by took them to Hôtel-Dieu.

Meanwhile, volunteers were streaming into the hospitals, including Grace, offering to help. They weren't turned away. A day later, *The Star* reported that "heroes (were) a dime a dozen" at the hospitals. The paper praised the city's population for its outreach.

The Star said "every doctor in the city phoned in offering his services, and firemen from Windsor had installed emergency lighting equipment so the operating rooms could be adequately lighted half an hour before it was needed."

Nurses labored through the rest of the day and night—some working 12 to 15 hours before picking up and going home. *The Star* reported, "Doctors half asleep as their feet slogged stubbornly along until the last casualty had been cleared." Meanwhile war veterans—themselves patients—vacated their beds and assisted nurses as they met the onslaught of new arrivals. They sat beside the battered and wounded, offering words of encouragement, or fetched pitchers of water.

As *The Star* reported, "the whole story is one of concerted unselfish effort." The reporter spun an account of one nurse who paused for a moment to get a breath of fresh air at an open doorway: " 'Sit down before you fall down, nurse,' said a waiting casualty seeing her stagger. 'I can't,' she said, and rushed back into the thick of it.' "

50th Anniversary Class—1946

The first, real "test" for these new nurses came two days after graduation in mid-June, when this devastating tornado turned Hôtel-Dieu upside down. Marian Page was one of 19 women from the 1946 graduating class, and that day she was still basking in a dream-come-true of being a nurse, and no longer in training. Then, suddenly, everything that she had studied came under abrupt scrutiny. The hospital's corridors were transformed into one large

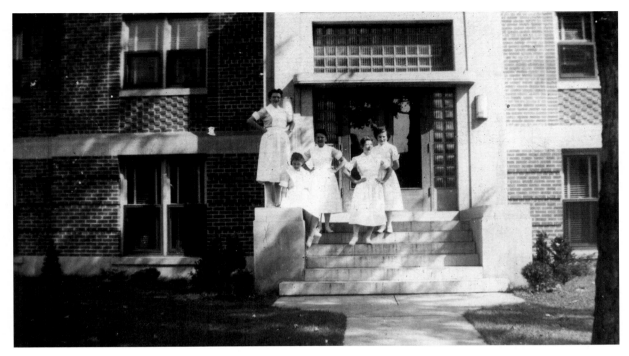

Nurses standing on the steps to the entrance of Hôtel-Dieu. (Courtesy of Freida Parker Steele)

emergency. Orderlies, nurses, doctors, police and firemen roamed the hallways dealing with the ever-mounting numbers being brought in from all over the city.

"That was our graduation gift," Page told *The Windsor Star* reporter.

In those early years, nurses worked 12-hour shifts, and they did this even when they were in training, but these did not include lectures that they had to attend. The students who worked the night shift had to rouse themselves from sleep in the afternoons, and go to class.

Staying out all night was not an option. The curfew set down by the sisters was 10 p.m.

The training in the 1940s was also different

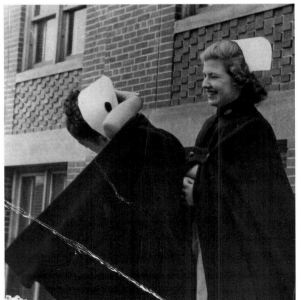

Nurses in front of Hôtel-Dieu

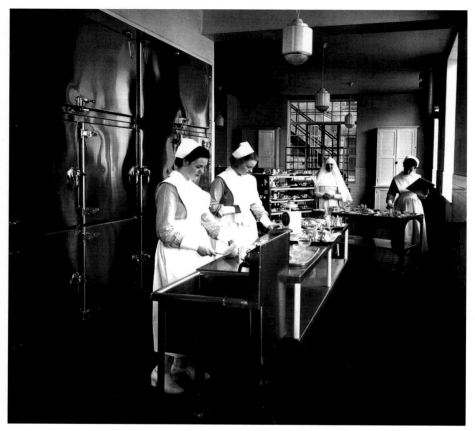

*Sister Claire Antaya
Supervisor, dietary and
students 1938*

patients when the buzzers are ringing off the wall, but they can't because of all the paperwork the government makes them do."

Sister Claire Antaya

She was 79 and still working. But her work was down the street from Hôtel-Dieu Hospital. She had discovered that a senior residence needed tending. Catholics there needed Holy Communion, a conversation, a pat on the back, some evidence that they were valued. Sister Antaya took it upon herself to do just that. Each and every day, she made her way a block down the street to Ouellette Manor where she was welcomed with open arms by the resident director.

Sister Antaya, a Eucharistic minister, knew that many of these elderly residents couldn't get out for mass. She saw her role as bringing them Holy Communion. In an interview, the kindly sister said, although it was a bit of chore, "every day (is) filled with new and often beautiful experiences." She said she was finally learning to listen. One lady confided in the sister that she hadn't seen anyone in two months, and that to prevent herself from going crazy, she read the paper out loud "to fill up the emptiness and not forget how to talk."

One day, when she was bringing Communion to a resident on the third floor—it was pre-arranged—she walked right into the apartment without knocking because she had been told to do that from the resident she was supposed to see. This, of course, was someone else's place—

from what was to follow. Marge O'Brien, in an interview with Chris Vander Doelen of the *Star* in July 1996 at the time of the 50th anniversary, said, "Today they have more book knowledge than we did. But we had more sympathy and compassion." The newspaper writer added, "Today's nurse…is hamstrung by bureaucracy, technology and malpractice insurance."

Marge McGuire, originally from Maidstone, was surprised at what nurses face today: "Lots of them would like to do more for the absolutely identical—and Sister Antaya realized this immediately, and apologized, and started to leave when the startled resident said, "Don't go away, sister, I just finished a novena to St. Anthony asking him to send someone to bring me Holy Communion, to visit me and—here you are. It is St. Anthony who sent you to me."

Antics at Jeanne Mance

How about the time an energetic young nursing student accidentally slid down a bannister into the convent and found herself in a sprawling meeting room lined with chairs and a long table in the centre? She quietly made her way through an unlocked door, and thought she hadn't been spotted. She had. There was hell to pay. Or the time another student posed as a mother-to-be and was rushed into the elevator in a wheelchair, and was about to be taken care of when she leapt from the chair in a nursing outfit that was under the heavy coat that she wore. Then there was that silly moment when two students came in late—long after curfew—and they were crawling on all fours. The night supervisor—a nun of course—spotted them, and asked, "Are you looking for something girls?"

The sisters took this all in good stride. They sensed some hooliganism would develop—it let off a little bit of steam. Minor disciplines were exacted from the student nurses, like mopping floors or cleaning out rooms. Make-work projects. Annoyances.

Polio

If you grew up in Windsor in the period after the Second World War and right up until the late 1950s, mothers would battle to keep their children at home, and out of the afternoon sun, but also away from outdoor splash pools, or the river. The scare was polio, your child falling ill with this crippling disease, and the scare was real. In 1946, nearly 10 years after the city was hit with the worst incidence of the disease, Paul Martin, Jr., who became Canada's prime minister in 2003, nearly died from it. It was late August 1946, and eight-year-old Paul and a buddy, Mike Maloney, were hanging out at the family cottage at Colchester. They had been swimming in Lake Erie and trading comic books and gorging themselves on fresh lake perch. The next morning when Paul awoke, he felt terribly ill. His neck was stiff and sore. He was also sick to his stomach. In an *Ottawa Citizen* article when Paul succeeded Jean Chrétien as Prime Minister, the writers quote Maloney as saying, "In those days, people were terrified of polio. It seemed like every year there would be an outbreak. And people would be walking in fear and trembling that their children were going to come down with it. And nobody knew where it came from."

Paul's mother, Nell, telephoned a doctor she knew, and he immediately suspected polio. Her son was rushed to Windsor by ambulance. Maloney told *The Ottawa Citizen*, "It was the kiss of death if somebody got polio."

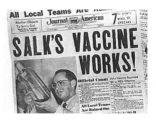

A breakthrough in the midst of the polio epidemic

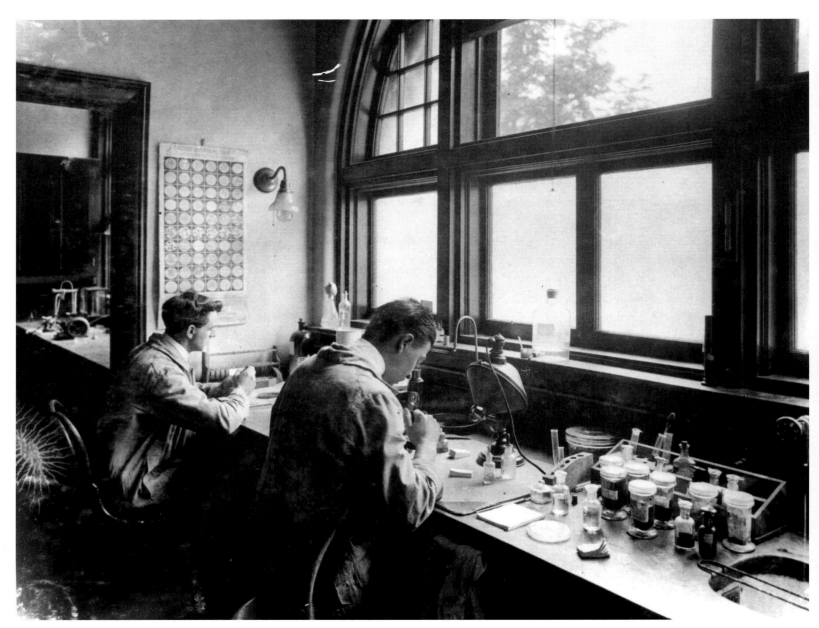

Orthopedic Lab, circa 1930s

At first, it was thought he should go to Hôtel-Dieu, but he wound up at Fred Adams' Isolation Hospital, or the annex that is now Metropolitan Hospital. In many instances, this was the routine. If there was any sign that the diagnosis might be polio, the sick were taken to the unit in South Walkerville. That day, Nell telephoned her husband, Paul Senior—then Secretary of State. He was in a federal cabinet meeting at the time. A messenger tiptoed into the meeting to tell him it was urgent, and that he should call his wife. The news stunned him, and when he slipped back into the meeting, he passed a note to Louis St. Laurent, then a fellow minister, who announced the news to the hushed room. Paul Martin returned home to his ailing son... For eight days, the family watched helplessly as their son lay there. Miraculously, the young Paul survived.

That story is not an isolated one. Poliomyelitis, or polio, hit Windsor like a sledgehammer nine years earlier in 1937, and again in 1939. Its first cases in Canada, however, were seen 10 years before that. In 1927 reports of it were coming from British Columbia, followed by Alberta, then Manitoba. In Ontario, there were occurrences as early as 1929. It was then referred to as "infantile paralysis." There was little research (partly because of the Great Depression) and limited funding, most of which was being spent on serums. In 1937, this started to change. It may have changed, too, because of Paul Martin himself. Christopher Rutty and

Sue C. Sullivan in *This Is Public Health: A Canadian History* note that Martin's father had had polio when he was a boy. That was in 1907. So when Paul Senior hopped that plane for Windsor, he knew the challenges of the disease. As the writers of this article suggest, "The interest of Ottawa in the polio problem grew…by the personal experience and political agenda of Paul Martin." But what confounded scientists and medical experts was that polio was now striking young adults too, not just children. Rutty and Sullivan quote A .R. Foley's article ("The Present Outbreak of Poliomyelitis in Quebec") from the *Canadian Public Health Journal* (Oct. 1932), as calling the disease "Death Walks In Summer." The magazine urged parents to be vigilant in watching their children and to "suspect everything" since no one could predict which case would prove mild or which would cripple hopelessly. By 1946, the advancements in research were still not where they might have been. The only real way to fight the disease was to use human "convalescent" serum made with blood collected from polio victims. The serum itself, however, had little effect on the paralytic effects of the disease. At least that was the assumption since those effects weren't discovered until the paralysis had already started. As with other diseases, the provincial authorities started issuing school closings and quarantines on public gatherings.

In 1946, when the young Paul Martin came down with polio, there seemed to be the same

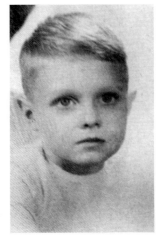

Future Prime Minister Paul Martin, Jr., was stricken with polio in 1946.

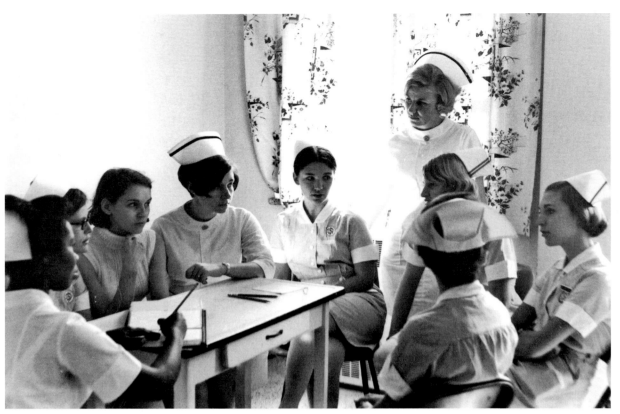

Instructors at Jeanne Mance Residence at a monthly meeting. The nurses up to the 1950s and 1960s wore the traditional caps and starched uniforms.

panic as there had been in a 1937 outbreak. The Fred Adams Isolation Hospital—a place named after and established by the former Medical Officer of Health for the city—was in full operation. But the polio record indicated that in 1941 there had been only six cases, three in 1942, none in 1943, 27 in 1944 (including two deaths), and seven cases in 1945. At the time Martin was at the hospital, 16 cases were being handled. But a 14-year-old boy had just died. The situation worsened. Total cases rose to 33, the highest in five years. Case loads were rising

across the country where authorities reported 594 cases. In Windsor, all the wading pools and beaches were shut down. The city's medical officer of health warned the public that the situation seemed "to be repeating what happened in 1937-39." In 1937, there had been 33 cases. Two years later, those numbers reached 48.

The big worry was the use of the respirator, or "iron lung." The thinking was that without the device, death was certain. The Fred Adams Hospital had only one iron lung and there was anxiety that if the power went out, it would shut off the respirator. The city thus started its search for an emergency unit.

In 1937, procedures of dealing with the disease were far less certain. Windsor didn't know how to handle it. Neither did other communities. Critics felt schools and public gatherings should be shut down, and people quarantined. Adams vehemently disagreed. His perspective was that if schools suddenly sent hundreds of kids home, there would be less control. Having them at school, and monitored, was far better. Adams said, "Closing schools is by no means a cure-all…It should be pointed out that when a child is at school he is in an airy room with plenty of space about him and under competent jurisdiction…I think very good school nurses and doctors are available in all our schools. I think the system can be trusted to send home any child who is in any degree suspicious."

This part of Southwestern Ontario, however, was clearly in panic mode in 1937. St. Anne's Church in Tecumseh drew 5,000 to its masses over the weekend for special prayers for miracles. A photograph of its pastor Rev. G. P. Pitre, appeared in the *Windsor Daily Star*. The priest had likened this effort to that of the famous Ste. Anne de Beaupre, Quebec where miracles had been reported.

The first "iron lung," constructed of huge metal cylinders that regulated the breathing of people whose polio attacked their respiratory muscles, was brought to Canada in 1930, and set up at Sick Children's Hospital in Toronto.

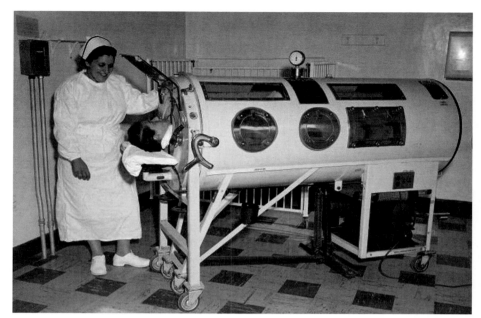

An iron lung brought to Toronto in 1930 made the rounds of the province.

In 1937, the flurry and rush to acquire more, sent the Ontario Government into a panic as it responded with an order for 27 in a six-week period.. Some women even gave birth while confined in an iron lung. The Royal Canadian Air Force also made emergency deliveries of these to different parts of the country. Windsor didn't get theirs until 1939. The device, however, was provincially owned and on loan to the city. It had been developed in 1937 to deal with the polio epidemic. More than 30 were manufactured at that time and the "lung" made the rounds in the province. In 1939, when there were virtually no episodes of polio, a lung was on loan to London. Adams had to requisition one for Windsor. At the same time, Adams—ever the diplomat—desperately tried to ratchet down the public

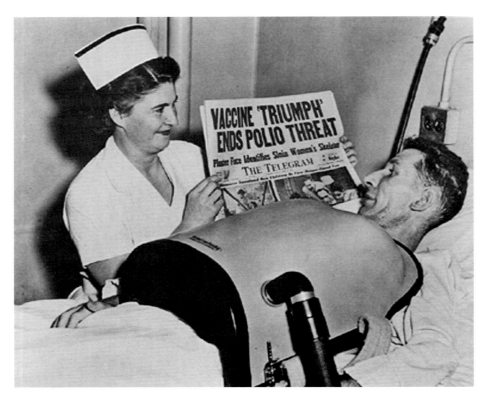

A nurse shows a polio patient the news of a vaccine.

For nearly thirty years, the writers quoted Jane S. Smith, the author of *Patenting the Sun: Polio and the Salk Vaccine*, as saying that polio was regarded "as a fierce monster that lurked in the damp hollows of (children's) experience," and was "a grim terror...more menacing, more sinister than death itself.'"

Hôtel-Dieu was on the edge of this, but its medical staff became acutely cognizant of the polio symptoms as people came through their doors looking for help. These were immediately dispatched to the Fred Adams Isolation Hospital, a five-minute drive across town.

Controversy over Nursing Graduates in 1950

It was June 1950. A moment to celebrate. A week before graduation. Forty-two young nurses from Hôtel-Dieu—eager to escape the watchful eyes of nuns and life in a hospital residence and get on with their lives -- decided to celebrate at the former Thomas' Inn on Riverside Drive.

Among the graduating class were two black nurses. In the midst of all their fun, these two young women were quietly escorted to the door, ordered to leave, and warned not to make a scene. It was Bertha Thomas, the legendary roadhouse owner, who explained to them she didn't want her other guests—white guests—to be disturbed. Freida Parker and Cecile Wright left without saying a word.

All hell broke loose, however, when Mayor

worry, but the numbers kept rising.

As an article issued from The Canadian Public Health Association explains, "no one knew if the disease was contagious or what could be done to prevent or treat it. Polio epidemics continued, usually in the summer or fall, and became more severe and affected older children and youth."

A cure for polio wasn't developed until the Salk and Sabine vaccines were introduced in 1955, and again in 1962. According to Rutty and Sullivan, the disease was one of the most feared of twentieth-century North America.

Art Reaume found out what happened—his own daughter was among the 42 nurses celebrating that night. What ensued was a flurry of press coverage, including columnist R.M. Harrison's scathing criticism of the hotel keeper—though never mentioning her name. He noted how ironic it was that, earlier, these same two black nurses had taken care of her when she had gone into the hospital and she didn't mind the treatment at all. Reaume told the press: "Let those who have been guilty of this most un-Christian act repent...."

Years later, Freida Parker Steele looks back at that event and smiles. Sure, it bothered her. Sure, it hurt. Sure, it made no sense. Sure, it was wrong. But she survived. Freida carries an air of self-confidence. She isn't one to be defeated. She has gone through life recognizing the "positives" and knows what it means to build on those. That's what the celebration was all about in 2000 when she, and other nurses, celebrated their 50th anniversary—coming together to party and chat about old times. Those impressionable years when they lived in residence at the Jeanne Mance building next door to the present Hotel-Dieu. It was there they worked side by side, rising at 5:30 a.m. to hot porridge and by 7 a.m. making breakfast for their patients. A day of running errands, cleaning rooms, making beds, scrubbing bed pans, folding linen, helping deliver babies, going to class...Three years of training. Cramming a lifetime into a lifetime.

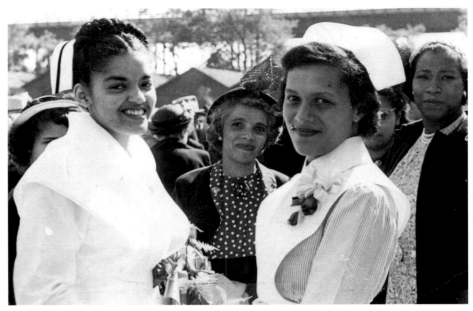

Freida Parker and Cecile Wright at graduation, 1950. (Courtesy of Freida Parker Steele)

Freida and Cecile weren't the first black nurses to graduate from Hôtel-Dieu. Two years before this in 1948, Colleen L. Campbell of Dresden, Ontario and Marian V. Overton of Windsor both graduated from the nursing program. The fight for black women to be permitted to take nursing training in Canada ended after the Second World War, according to Peggy Bristow in her article "A Duty to the Past, A Promise to the Future: Black Organizing in Windsor" published in *The Journal of Black Canadian Studies* (New Dawn, Vol. 2, No. 1, 2007).

Freida and Montreal-born Cecile Wright graduated together in 1950, but it was Wright who received the headlines in a black newspaper, published in Windsor. The headline read

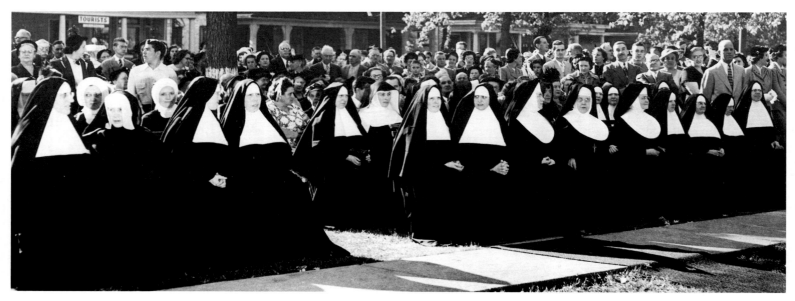

Opening of the 1952 wing

"Cecile Wright Earns New Honors for Race." Both black girls, however, sailed through the three years without fuss. They were eagerly received by their classmates and, like them, they were steeped in all the craziness of it.

Freida remembers someone meticulously stenciling the words *St. John's Toilet Paper* on each roll of toilet paper for the St. John wing of Hôtel-Dieu, the wing reserved for Windsor's VIPs. And someone else patching rubber gloves or sharpening the syringes. Or students spying for the nuns on the doctors to make sure they didn't do tubal ligation on women of child-bearing age. Or the fainting in the Operating Room, as Pat Mowat did, and then being grilled by the nuns who wanted to know if she was pregnant. Pregnancy during training was grounds for dismissal.

> *"Working in a hospital...They learned to see goodness in all that seemed hopeless."*

There were also moments of sadness and the hearts of these young students went out to the 16-year-old girls who died after hemorrhaging from "back alley abortionists." Or to the young prostitutes brought in by the ambulance drivers. Win (Auld) Sinclair recalled how they were treated with utmost respect by the nuns. It opened their eyes. This slice of life. Working in a hospital where they witnessed families dealing with death, children fighting for their lives, women down and out, eager and hopeful for a better future. It opened the eyes of these 42 nurses. It shaped their lives. It shaped the way they looked at the world. They learned not to judge. They learned to accept people for who they were. They learned to see goodness in all that seemed hopeless.

As Freida recalled, there was the time she

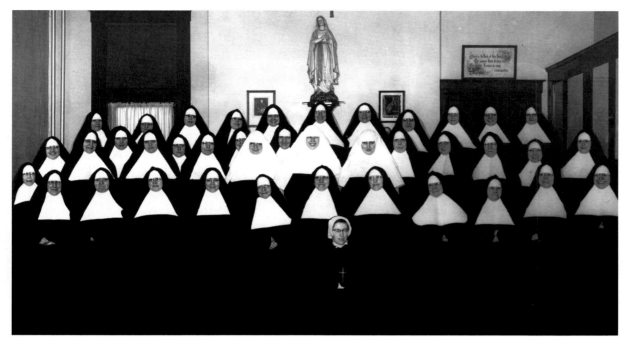

In 1953, the Sisters at Hôtel-Dieu were still the dominant force behind the operation of their hospital. All of that would gradually change.

enjoined her mom to make some ginger bread for the street people, all the homeless and alcoholics, on the second floor ward. It was her father, Al Parker, a police detective, who brought these sweets in for her to distribute to these patients.

"I told him what nice people they all were, but when he stepped into the room, he recognized all but one -- he had arrested them all at one time or another."

The other thing about that class of 1950? The lesson that was never taught. Genie (Denomme) Van Hooren said it was the cement of friendship, the loyalty, the camaraderie born on the very day they met 50 years ago. It survived everything.

The Superiors

Sister Claire Maître

Claire grew up on a small farm at the outskirts of Tecumseh, where her father also worked as a carpenter. School was two miles down the road, and this was long before there were school buses. The children set out in the early morning to make it to class on time. Claire had considered becoming a teacher but she was held back, having to care for her three younger sisters at home. Claire's mother was a sickly woman, and needed her to fill in where she could not. Throughout this time, Claire fixed her attention on the future, and her vocation. As she states in her own written notes,

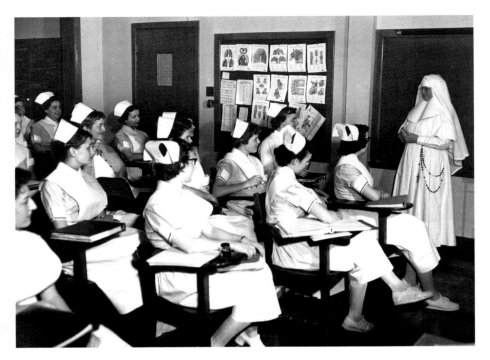

Sister Claire Maître teaches a class at Hôtel-Dieu's School of Nursing

she found the time to pray in private—not on her knees, but while doing the farm chores, or tending to her siblings.

"My prayers became intense. I prayed everywhere, anywhere, not always kneeling," Claire said. Then again, family prayer was something that had been fostered in the Maître family. As her notes attest, "If visitors came at prayer time, they were expected to kneel and join in. No exceptions were allowed." Meanwhile, Claire's mother provided detailed catechism lessons. She also told them Bible stories.

At age 13 and again at age 17, following her mother's death, Claire asked her father for permission to enter the convent. According to her notes, this proved to be the "wrong time." The parish priest sided with her father's disapproval, and told her she was too young. Claire continued to help out at home, but also started earning some money by cleaning houses in the neighbourhood.

Claire's life changed when she went to live with an uncle in St. Lambert, Quebec. This uncle was married to a woman who was often ill, and needed assistance with his four young children. It was while she was in Quebec that Claire developed an even greater attraction to the religious life. Again she was knocking on the doors of the religious community at St. Joseph's Oratory at Mount Royal. The Superior turned her away, advising her to return home, "make friends, and have a good time and then re-think" this vocation.

In 1918, the Spanish Flu spread across the country, and Claire's older brother, returning from the war, died suddenly. He was 24. So did her Aunt Emily from St. Lambert. She also lost two sisters. By 1920, Claire had decided it was time to return to Tecumseh. She was looking for work with a family, perhaps a mother with small children—a mother who might be ill, as hers had been. Claire wrote down her feelings in a diary: "It is here I began to perceive that my own wishes seemed to have changed. Having cared for so many sick people, and learned so much about nursing, that career appealed to me more than any other. After making the rounds of the religious communities, I finally decided to register for the nursing course at Hôtel-Dieu Hospital School of Nursing and enter the convent."

It was Mother Marie de la Ferre who first spoke to Claire about the order. She was the Superior at the time. In October 1924, Claire entered the Windsor convent. Sister Maria Guevin was the Mistress of Novices, and she inspired and encouraged Claire, and assigned her to be the local secretary of the community. She also filled in other departments, including radiology, the pharmacy and the lab. In 1929, Claire graduated from the School of Nursing. She also made her final vows to become Sister Maître. This occurred a year after the death of her father. She cared for him in his final days and, according to her biographers, this proved to be valuable because the rift that had existed between the two was reconciled. According to the story, Claire's father had always resented his daughter's interference in a family matter that involved another one of her sisters. That altercation resulted in her father telling Claire to leave the house. That's when she went to live with her uncle. Claire and her father, however, finally resolved their differences.

By 1933, it was clear the School of Nursing needed someone of Sister Claire Maître's expertise. She leapt at the opportunity, but meanwhile pursued acquiring a Bachelor of Arts Degree from the University of Western Ontario in 1937. Her ambition didn't stop there. She then acquired a Bachelor of Science of Nursing Education in London, Ontario. By 1942, Sister Maître was administrator of Hôtel-Dieu, but also continued training nurses at the hospital's school. She was responsible for the opening of the Jeanne Mance School of Nursing; it would operate until 1973 when the provincial government ordered all such training to be done at community colleges.

"Sister Maître was a sturdy woman, and she had strong character. She was also pretty straight with the nurses, especially to the girls who were from out of town. She was more motherly to us (the novices)," said Sister Cecile LeBoeuf, who would later become Superior of Windsor's Religious Hospitallers.

Sister Maître ceased working at Hôtel-Dieu in 1947 when a job opened up for her in Northern Alberta at Whitelaw. In 1979, she returned to Hôtel-Dieu. In October 1992 she had a terrible fall one morning in the chapel at Villa Maria, and never fully recovered. Sister Maître died 11 days before Christmas 1995.

Sister Blanche Garceau

Blanche grew up on a farm near Verner, Ontario. She came from a large family. She had five sisters and two brothers. At six, she nearly drowned when she tumbled into a creek near the farm. She was rescued by one of her sisters. She often told people she was meant to live—there was a purpose for her. Blanche, in telling the story, quoted Isaiah (43:2): "I am certain

God was watching over me." Indeed, a few years later, the farmhouse her family lived in burned to the ground. Then her mother's health began to fail, and Blanche's schooling had to be "curtailed," say the convent's biographers. It was just before her mother's death that Blanche announced her decision to become a nun. She wrote, "I remember telling her that I would like to become a nun, and she didn't seem to think that I would ever make the grade." The following spring—1925—Blanche's mother passed away. That's when Blanche moved to Windsor. She wanted to join her married sisters and find work. For four years, she tasted the world of the city, playing sports, going to dances and dating. In December 1929, she finally entered the Religious Hospitallers of St. Joseph. It hadn't been her dream. As a child, she had always seen herself as a teacher, but somehow the two occupations came together in one. In 1943, Sister Garceau shared the responsibility of teaching in Hôtel-Dieu's School of Nursing. She also received her Bachelor of Science from the University of St. Louis. From 1944 to 1947, Sister Garceau acted as Mistress of the Novices, and then was appointed Superior, and in 1950 was made Hospital Administrator. Like her predecessors, she would step down and take over the running of Villa Maria, and much later the directorship of Jeanne Mance School of Nursing.

It came as a surprise to her, but in 1970 she was sent to be the Superior of the order at Whitelaw, Alberta. In 1977, however, she re-

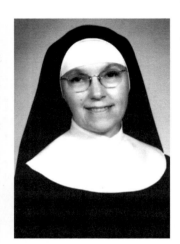

Sister Blanche Garceau, 1965

turned to Windsor, due to ill health. Soon she was placed in charge of pastoral care at Hôtel-Dieu. Sister Garceau passed away in 2001. As her biographers say:

"Sister Blanche humbly accepted the limitations and frailty of age and health; and her smile was contagious. Her sense of community did not diminish, however, and she expressed her gratitude to be able to join the community in evening prayer in the community room. At this stage, her participation was one of listening, since her failing eyesight did not permit reading anymore. However, she could be heard singing, praying the parts she knew from memory after so many years spent in prayer."

Sister Rose Anna Tétrault

In April 2013, Sister Tétrault turned 104. She died in July 2013. Behind her was much of the history of the religious order that she joined in 1931. She had made the decision to become a nun, knowing it would disappoint many in her family. The 22-year-old Rose, whose life had been put on hold because of her mother's ill health, and finally her passing away, decided she would join three other women to enter the convent in November 1931. In a way, it was made easier for her with three others accompanying her. In her autobiographical notes, Sister Tétrault writes:

"The four of us crossed from the hospital to the cloister thinking we would never again leave the community, never return home, see our families only rarely and lead a life of sacrifice useful to the salvation of the world and our personal sanctification. This did not scare me."

Sister Tétrault grew up five miles east of Tilbury in St. Francis Xavier parish. Her family was staunchly Catholic. "We said our morning and night prayers at my mother's knee when we were small and continued to do this by ourselves as we grew up. We prayed the rosary and certain litanies in common." Problems, however, arose in school where the priest taught them catechism, and she and her siblings struggled with this because they spoke only French. Sister Tétrault had planned on entering the School of Nursing in Chatham, but with her mother's death, she had to take care of her family—a father and four brothers. "Fortunately, I had started to drive the car at 16 at my mother's suggestion. This helped me a great deal," she wrote. The tug to become a nun had always been with her. Even at five, Sister Tétrault recalls following her Aunt Lucie, a Catholic nun, all around the house on one of her visits. "I remember being asked the usual question as to what I would do when I grew up. The answer came spontaneously: I would be a nun like her." Sister Tétrault recalls discussing this possibility with her mother, but her mother discouraged her daughter. "She would answer,

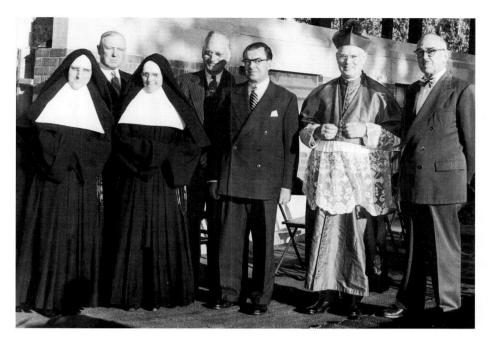

Sr. Rose Anna Tétrault, Sr. Blanche Garceau, Chairman of the Board Anthony Fuerth, Contractor Cleveland Mousseau, Hon. Paul Martin, Bishop Cody of London Diocese, Architect James Pennington at the laying of the cornerstone for the new 1952 wing of Hôtel-Dieu

'I don't think you are pious enough. You are not as prayerful as your sister.'" To that end, Sister Tétrault started "applying herself," as she said: "We had a beautiful print of the Sacred Heart in the guestroom downstairs where I would stop occasionally to say a prayer as the Holy Spirit inspired me."

Finally, as Sister Tétrault explained, she became "a realist." Her biggest worry was her father's reaction to her desire to be a nun. But he surprised her: He told her, "If you think you have a religious vocation, I certainly will not stand in the way." This approval came as a huge relief to all Sister Tétrault's wrangling over whether this was the right course of action. Her teachers in the novitiate were Sister

Guevin and Sister Marie de la Ferre. In 1933, she made her temporary vows. For a brief period, she had to return to finish high school and study at St. Mary's Academy before being admitted to Hôtel-Dieu's School of Nursing. Afterwards, both she and Sister Blanche Garceau were sent to Detroit to do postgraduate studies at Women's Hospital. This was followed by yet more studies, this time at St. Louis University in Missouri where Sister Tétrault received her Bachelor of Science in nursing education. She was surprised when she returned in 1943 and immediately was appointed the hospital's director. Seven years later, in 1950, she was made Superior at Hôtel-Dieu. In her time in the convent, so said *The Windsor Star*, she saw the hospital grow from a 125-bed institution to 450 beds. During her time as Superior, Hôtel-Dieu built itself a new school of nursing. The sisters were graduating two classes every year.

Soon, Sister Tétrault found herself immersed in the politics of the Sisters of Religious Hospitallers. The various congregations, both in Canada and the U.S., were struggling to form one centralized congregation. This had been talked about for years, and if it formed, it would mean the "houses" would be grouped into provinces. The decision to proceed with this resulted in the predominantly French-speaking Windsor congregation having to make a choice. The sisters at Hôtel-Dieu took a vote, and theirs was to go with the Montreal

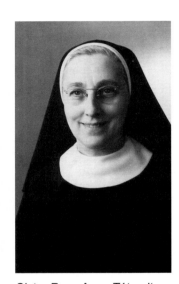

Sister Rose Anna Tétrault

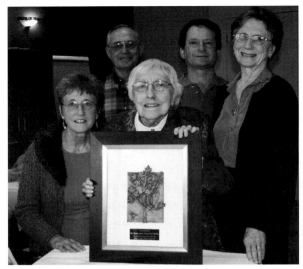

Sister Tétrault with her plaque and family

congregation, not Kingston. Much to Sister Tétrault's surprise, she was asked to be one of the general councilors of this new organization. It would mean moving to Montreal. She was appointed Assistant General: "I felt so unworthy, so ill-prepared, so lacking in the talents and know-how to fulfill such an important position. The Lord knows what it cost me to pack up and leave my dear community of Windsor." Over time, Sister Tétrault would become the General Superior of this new governing body of the sisters.

In her autobiographical statement, Sister Tétrault looked back at her life, and wrote this:

"With my 80th birthday fast approaching, it happens that I look back at my past life ...After such a full life, there remains a feeling of uncertainty. What have I really done all these years that is really pleasing to God and totally selfless? My hands feel empty! Must I return to the Maker having accomplished so little?"

Sister Viola Beaulieu

Viola Beaulieu's biographers say that when she passed away in 2003, the community knew they would miss "her beautiful smile, her teasing and her beautiful singing voice." She was 90, having been born in St. Joachim, Ontario. She made her final vows in 1937 and was made Supervisor of the surgical floor. She didn't graduate as a nurse until 1940. In 1950, Sister Beaulieu became Mistress of the Novices, and in 1953 took over as Superior of Hôtel-Dieu, and remained so until 1959. At this point, Sister Beaulieu was sent to Montreal where she served as assistant to the Provincial Superior until 1971. Like others, she also went to Whitelaw and served as its Superior.

In 1979, she returned to Hôtel-Dieu to assist in the infirmary and serve as Superior of Villa Maria. Her life had been full, and it became clear that Sister Beaulieu would never have been content to embrace it any other way. She met each day with new enthusiasm and her presence imbued that spirit into the community around her. For one, she was a practical joker, and loved to target the most serious of those around her—all in the name of bringing those

individuals down to reality. She once surprised a visiting priest with the quip: "Well, you know … we all need to be forgiven!" And when her memory was failing, Sister Beaulieu knew what age had brought to her awareness and memory, and at one point on a document, she purposely, and with some humour, scrawled, "My memory is failing—forgetful—I wrote this May 3, 1997."

In another instance, realizing her mind had been slipping, she once informed an inquiring and caring sister in the infirmary that she was fine—she was just using her imagination in a more creative way. "I'm just travelling right now," she said with a knowing smile.

Another Hôtel-Dieu sister quoted in the biographical notes left behind said this of Sister Beaulieu: "When we think of her, we recall her welcoming smile, her gentleness, her sense of humour and her kindness." In another folder just before she died, she left this note: "My will—My vows are in my trunk. Bye! God love you all. I do."

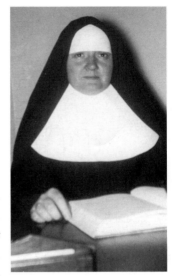

Sister Viola Beaulieu

Sister Germaine Lafond

Sister Germaine Lafond was born in 1899 in Sainte-Scholastique, Quebec, now just a stone's throw away from Mirabel Airport. She passed away in November 1975 after two massive heart attacks. Her biographers say, however, that her death was not expected because, throughout her life, she experienced many health setbacks and always returned with renewed zest to tackle the work in her community. When she died, the sisters stated that her passing had "thrown consternation on the motherhouse."

Sister Lafond's early education was with the sisters at Pensionnat des Soeures de Sante-Croix. From there, she was drawn to join the Hôtel-Dieu sisters in Montreal. She entered the convent in August 1921. As her biographers point out, there was no fretting over her vocation. "She was well aware of it, and was willing to fight and march strong with a free spirit to take her vows." This took place in 1923, almost two years to the day that she entered the cloister. When the sisters reflect on her contributions, they remember her as "la batisseuse" or "the builder." Her first assignment was working in the ophthalmic clinics, but also in surgery, and she spent long nights at the bedside of the sick. She fell gravely ill with a lung infection in 1930 and nearly died. When she returned to work, Sister Lafond was assigned as the hospital's dietician, a position she never felt comfortable with because it was an area she knew little about. To allay her worries, Sister Lafond threw herself into its study and became a valuable resource to the hospital and her community.

Nine years after her illness, the sister found herself tackling yet another area that she felt as beyond her reach, but it would serve as the foundation for the future developments at Hôtel-Dieu in Windsor, Ontario. Sister Lafond became the order's financial officer. Her keen insights led to her election as Assistant Gen-

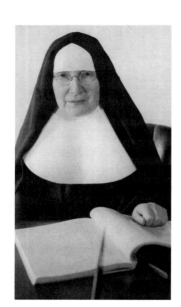

Sister Germaine Lafond was called affectionately 'Mere Canadienne.'

eral of Hôtel-Dieu, Montreal. Her biographers said: "She takes her new role as a leader with calmness and serenity." Her work there also resulted in building a new home-hospital in nearby (to Montreal) Sainte-Catherine. She didn't stay long. Soon she was founding the first mission of nurse-nuns of Saint Joseph in an urban village located north of Dahomey, 200 miles from Porto-Novo, now the official capital of the West African nation of Benin. It had been the capital of French Dahomey when Sister Lafond was there. Her foundation sent in nuns to help and train others, and urge the community to build a hospital servicing the needs of newborns in a clinic and an ambulance station. Sister Lafond was so well loved that villagers called her "Mère Canadienne."

In Windsor, Sister Lafond served as Superior from 1959 to 1965. She oversaw major renovations to the hospital, the construction of the chapel, and the building of a new convent. She was also there to oversee construction of a new wing to Hôtel-Dieu and the removal of the original 1888 structure. When she stepped down from her job of running the hospital, she continued to be on its planning committee with the idea of drawing up blueprints for the new hospital. "She is very respected amongst the workers for her experience with the different buildings that she worked on," state her biographers. They said she brought insight and practicality to the business of what was needed for the future, both for the hospital and the convent.

Saluting Our Doctors

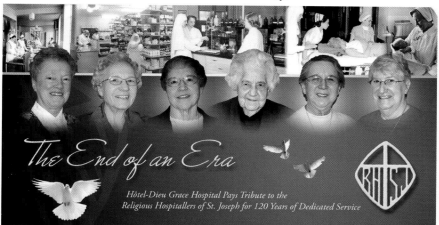

Hôtel-Dieu Grace Hospital Celebrates National Doctors' Day

2011, bulletin poster celebrates national Doctors' Day.

The End of an Era

Hôtel-Dieu Grace Hospital Pays Tribute to the Religious Hospitallers of St. Joseph for 120 Years of Dedicated Service

Bulletin poster celebrates the 120th anniversary of Hôtel-Dieu Grace Hospital and the hard work that staff has put in over the years.

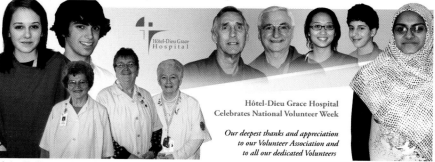

Hôtel-Dieu Grace Hospital Celebrates National Volunteer Week

Our deepest thanks and appreciation to our Volunteer Association and to all our dedicated Volunteers

A bulletin poster showing thanks to volunteers at Hôtel-Dieu Grace Hospital.

Photo Gallery

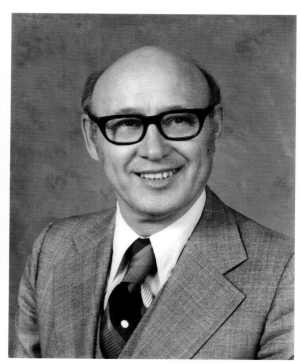

Roman Mann, Executive Director at Hôtel-Dieu from 1968 to 1990

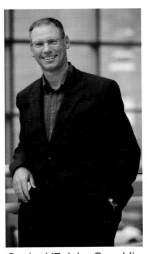

Senior VP John Coughlin of HDGH

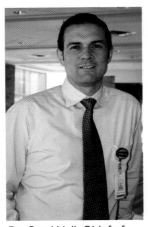

Dr. Gord Vail, Chief of Staff, 2010

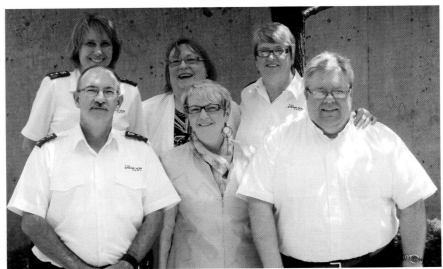

Chaplains, 2011: back row, Major Linda Daley, Olivia Hefner, Violet Chaulk front row, Major Steve Daley, Pat Slavik, Fr. Chris Bourdeau

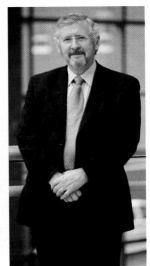

Sister Cecile LaBoeuf

Neil McEvoy, former Hôtel-Dieu Grace CEO

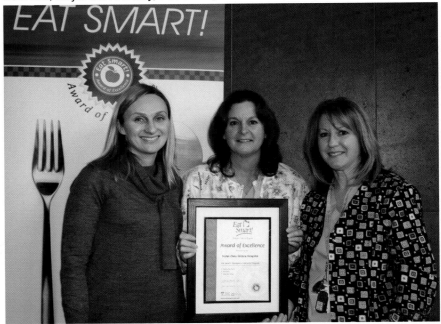

EatSmart Award Presentation 2010: Sarah Baker, Windsor Essex Health Unit presents award to Karen Skeates and Mary Schmidt

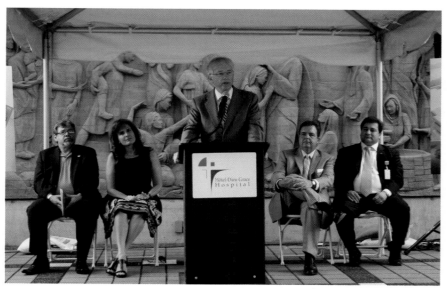

Ken Deane, Angioplasty announcement, 2011

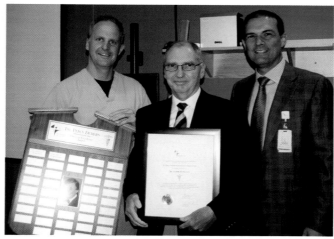

Dr. Frank DeMarco, centre, receives the Percy Demers Award for Physician Excellence, 2013

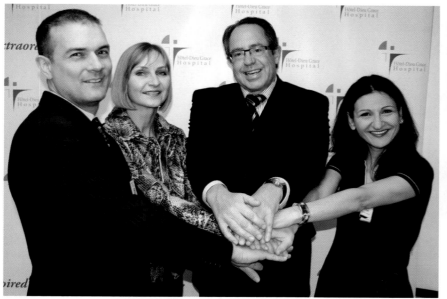

Doctors' Day, 2011: Dr. Gord Vail, Dr. Brigitte Ala, Dr. Bill Taylor and Dr. Sophia Thomas

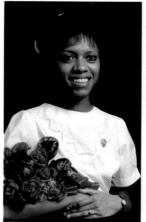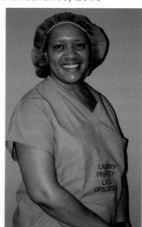

Barb Porter in her nursing graduation photo, left, and as an Operating Room Nurse

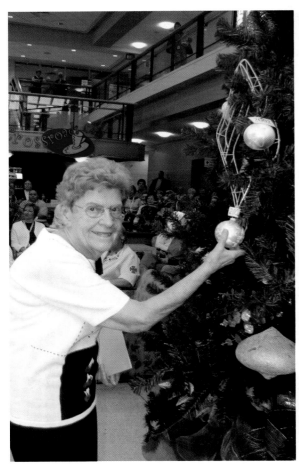

Eunice Sinclair with the Tree of Lights, 2005

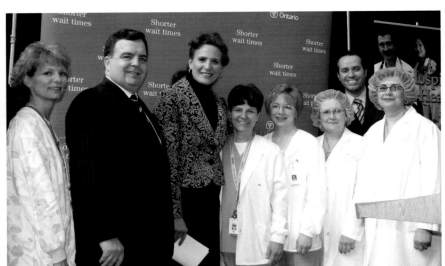

April 27, 2004, MPPs Dwight Duncan and Sandra Pupatello at HDGH

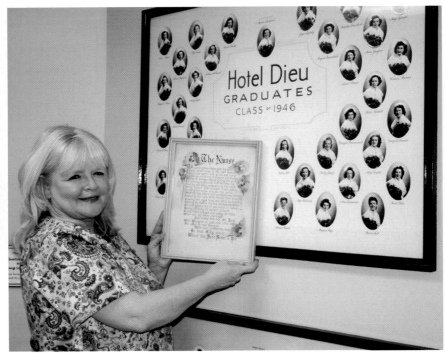

Maureen Guinard Renal Satellite, 2011, at her mother's graduating class photo

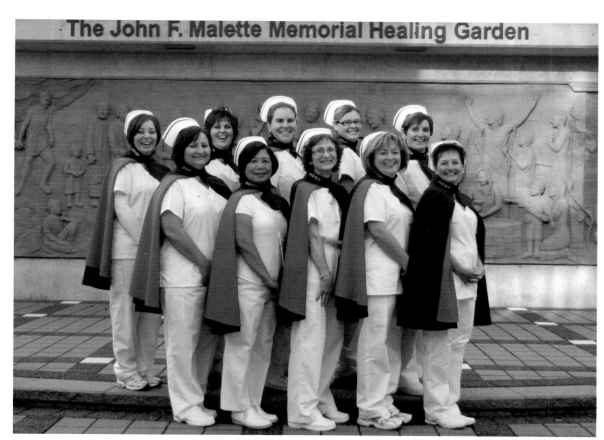

ER Nurses Honour Guard

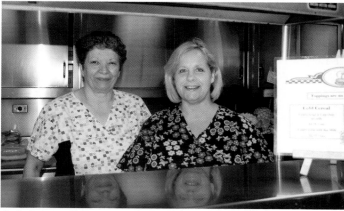

Cafeteria staff Rosa Del Percio and Cindy Viselli

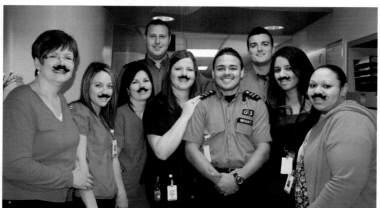

Movember, 2012

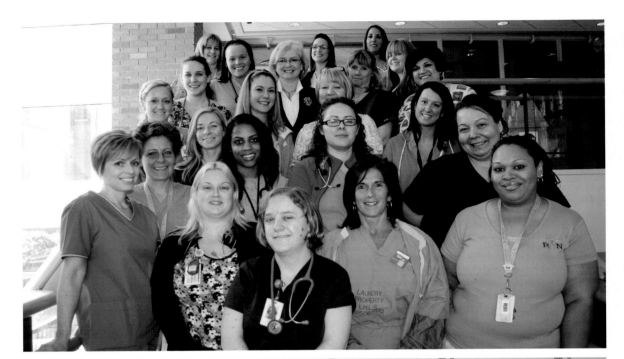

Nurses Week Windsor Star ad, 2012

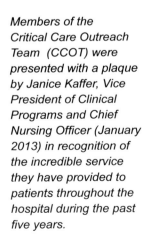

Members of the Critical Care Outreach Team (CCOT) were presented with a plaque by Janice Kaffer, Vice President of Clinical Programs and Chief Nursing Officer (January 2013) in recognition of the incredible service they have provided to patients throughout the hospital during the past five years.

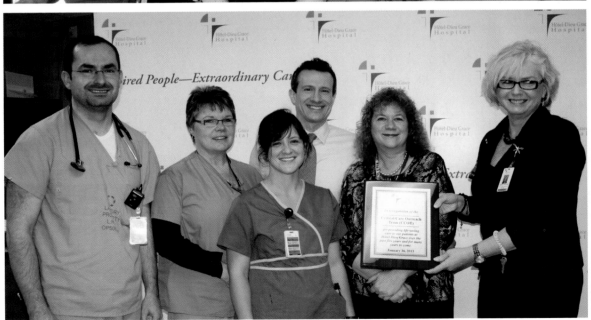

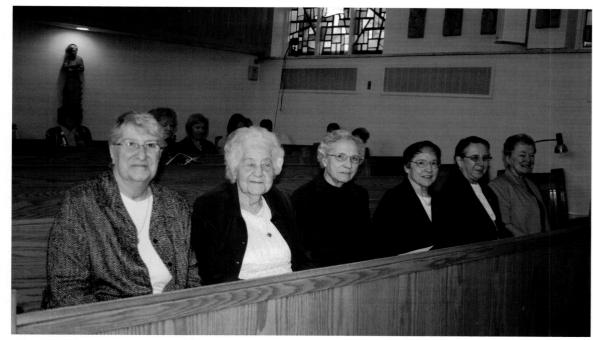

Six Sisters in Chapel, March 27, 2009, left to right: Sr. Angelina Duguay, Sr. Cecile LeBoeuf, Sr. Aurore Beaulieu, Sr. Marguerite Laporte, Sr. Bernice Bondy, Sr. Rose-Marie Dufault

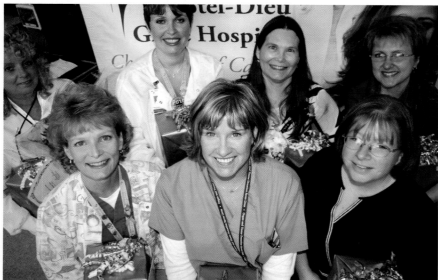

Nurses Week, 2008: Jeanne Mance Nursing Excellence Award recipients

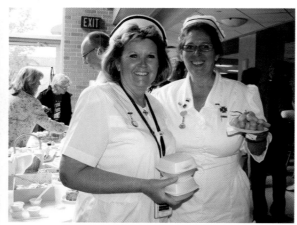

Nurses Week, 2012: Barb Mingay and JoDee Brown show off their white uniforms and nurses caps

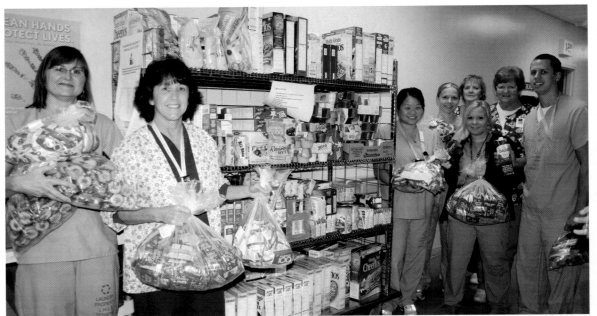

*Diagnostic Imaging
Staff collect food for the
Downtown Mission*

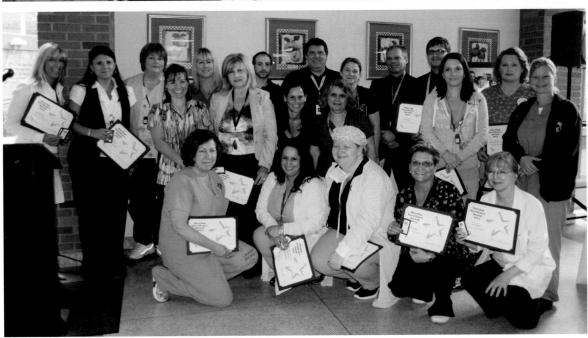

*Nursing Excellence
Awards, 2012*

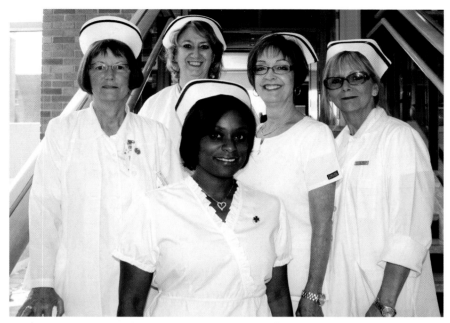

Nurses pose in their white uniforms, 2013

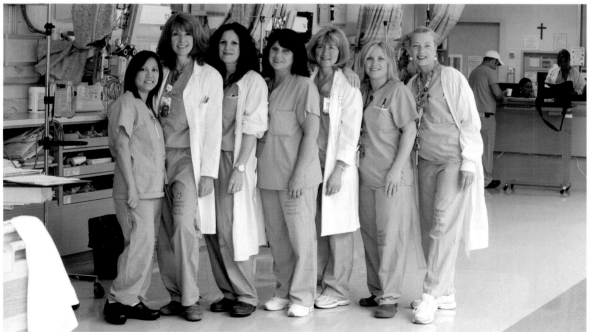

Post-Anesthesia Care Unit Staff

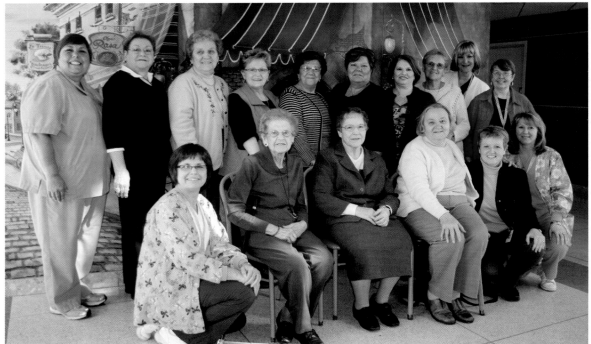

Sister Laporte (centre) farewell from Nutrition Services, 2009

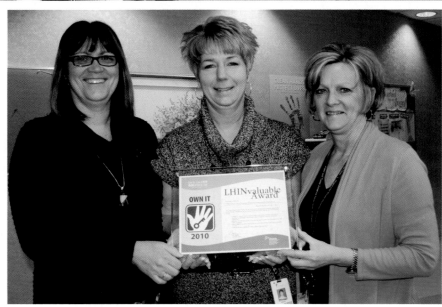

Renal Dialysis Staff Debbie Hodgins, Angie Tuovinen and Paula Bonelli pose with the LHIN OWN IT Award, 2010

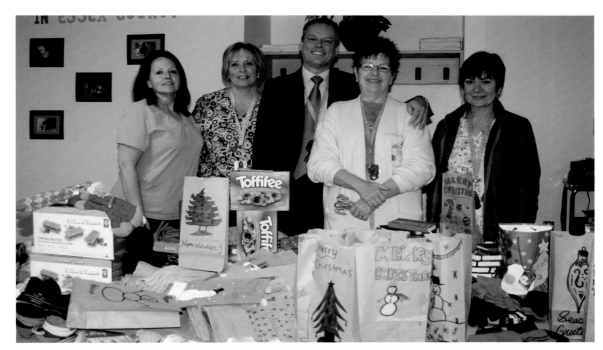

The Mental Health staff prepare Christmas bags for patients, 2011

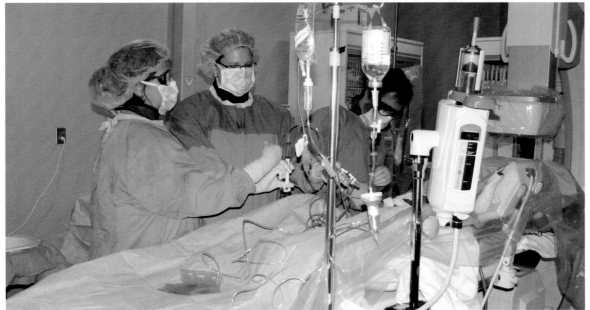

Cardiac Catheterization Lab

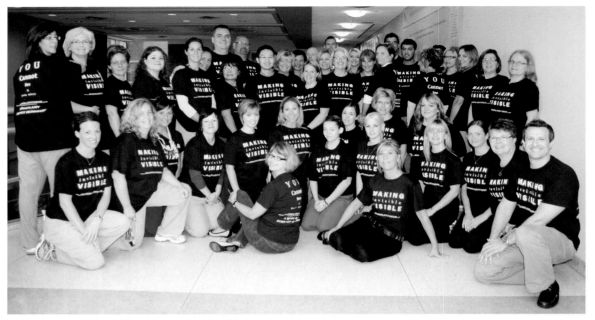

Staff and physicians posed for a photograph wearing their 'Making Invisible Visible' t-shirts for a bulletin board to celebrate Brain Injury Month in June, 2012

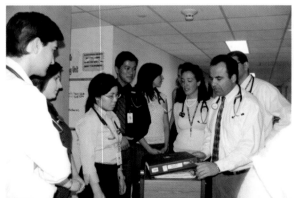

CTU Rounds with Dr. Tarabain, 2006. (Clinical Teaching Unit)

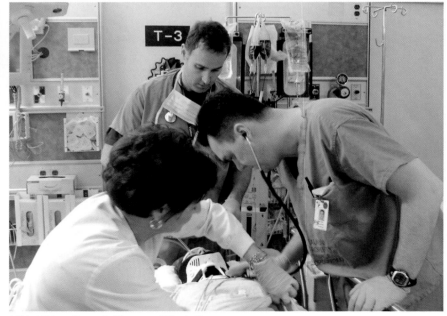

Hôtel-Dieu Grace's Trauma ER staff

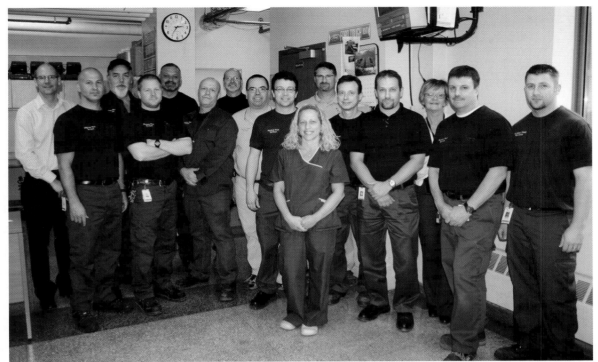

Physical Plant Staff, 2012

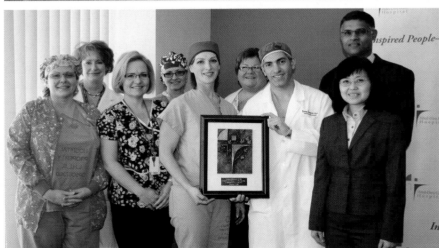

February 8, 2013, Dr. Emara and cataract surgery team presented with an award for excellence

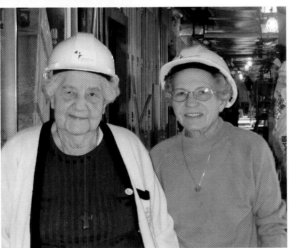

Sister Cecile LeBoeuf and Sister Beaulieu on a Hôtel-Dieu Grace construction site

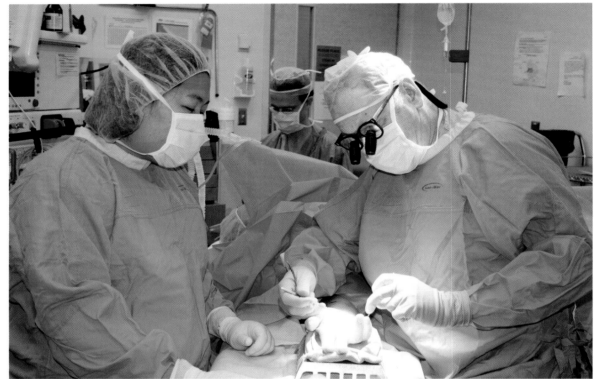

Operating Room, Dr. Adams

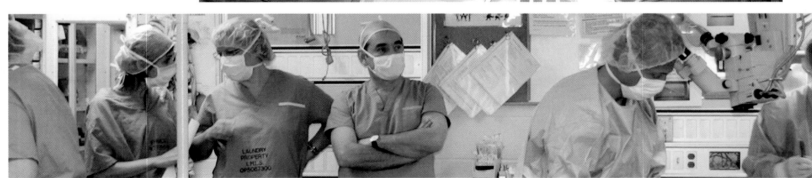

Operating room staff at work

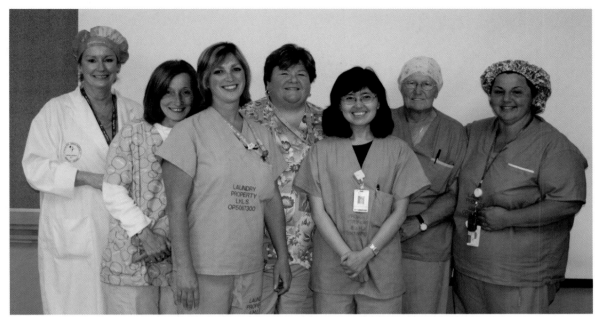

Dr. Ann Chiu and the Corneal Transplant Team, 2009

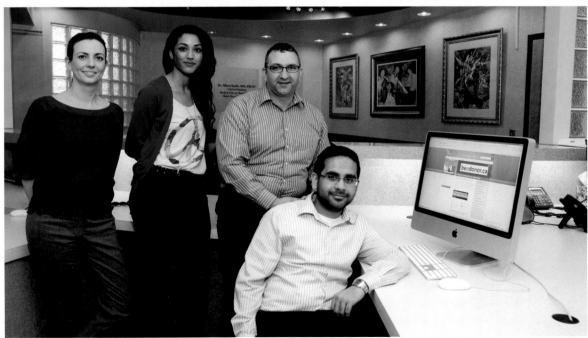

Dr. Al Kadri and team at the Renal Clinic, 2013

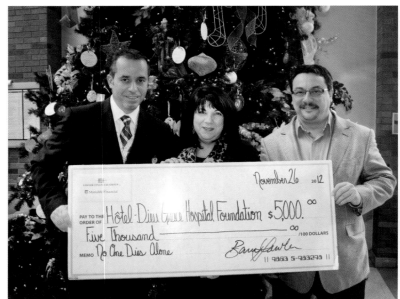

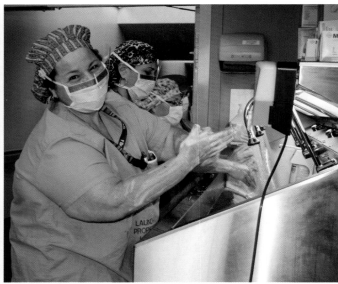

Registered Nurse First Assistants scrubbing for surgery, 2010

Bill Marra, President and Executive Director of HDGH Foundation, and Maria Giannotti, HDGH Pastoral Services, received a $5,000 cheque from Barry Fowler, President of Fowler Financial Group, to support the No One dies Alone program at the hospital

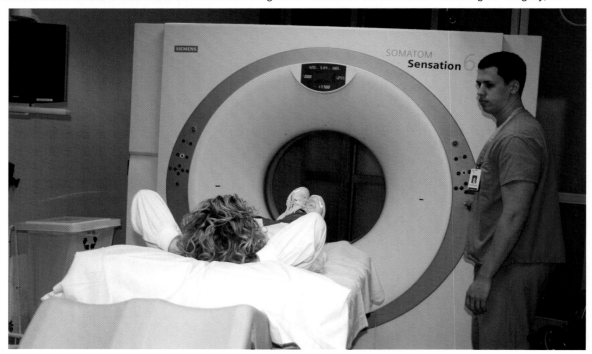

The new 64 Slice CT

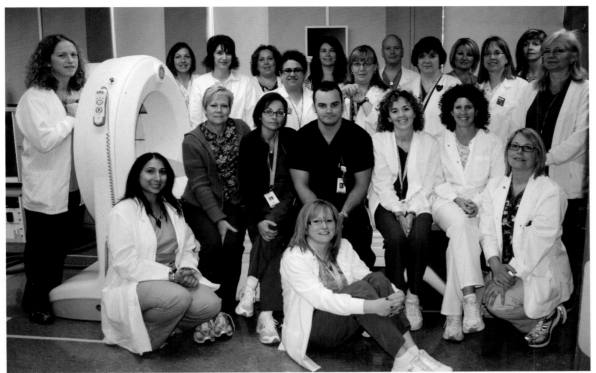

The Nuclear Medicine team, 2009

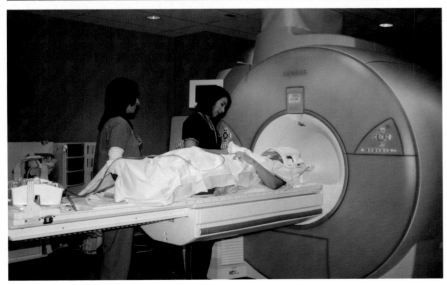

The new MRI, 2008

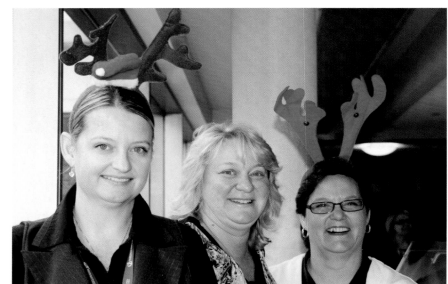

Christmas Luncheon, 2009, Health Records Staff

8-East Christmas, 2009

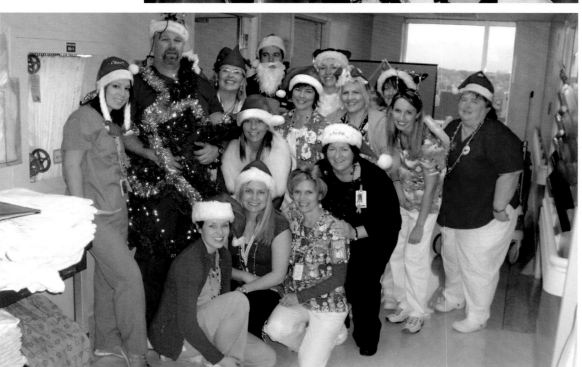

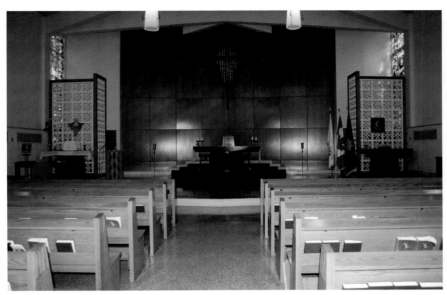

2010, Hôtel-Dieu Grace's chapel

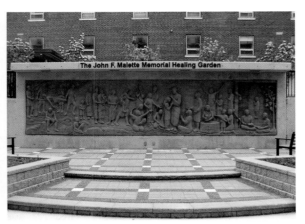

Malette Garden - healing garden

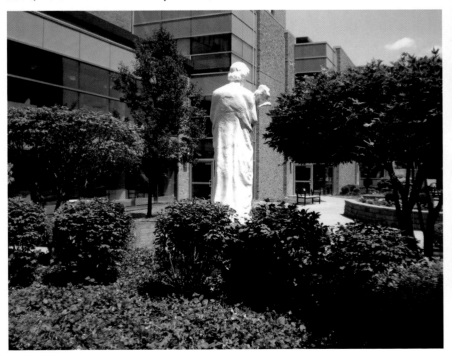

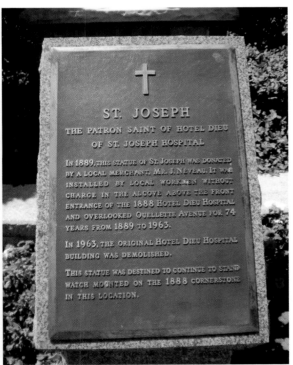

Plaque near the statue of St. Joseph (left) which was mounted on the 1888 cornerstone when the original Hôtel-Dieu Hospital was demolished in 1963

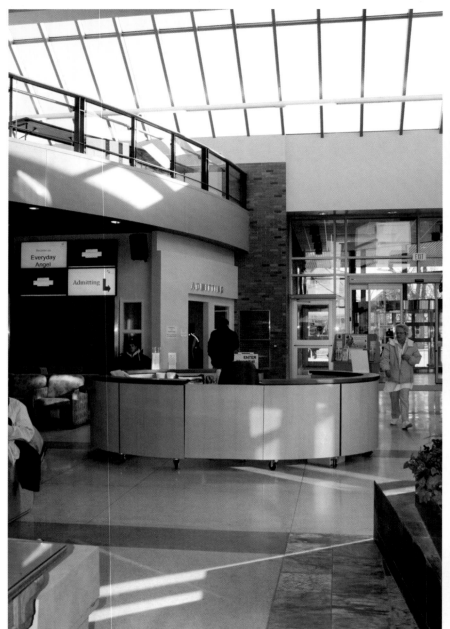

The lobby for the Goyeau entrance of HDGH

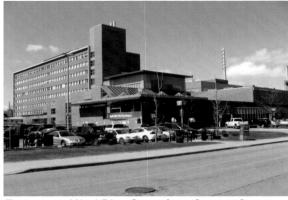

Entrance to Hôtel-Dieu Grace from Goyeau Street

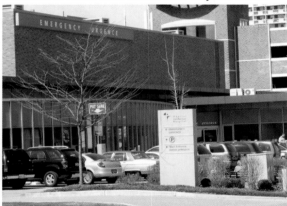

Goyeau view of HDGH

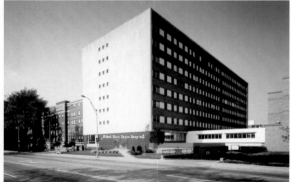

Ouellette Entrance to HDGH

PART IV

A New Generation

1960s-1970s

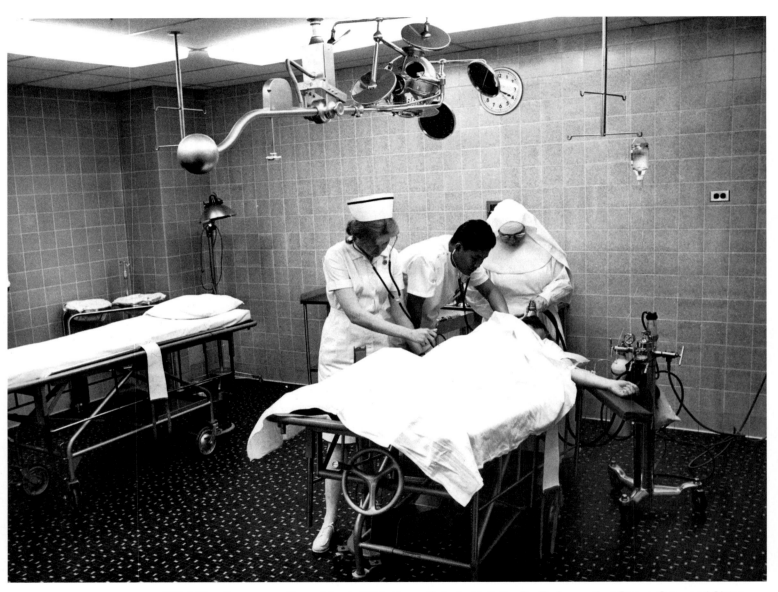

Hôtel-Dieu Emergency Room March 1964. Nurse Celeste Mellotte, Dr. Enrico, patient Donna Gray, and Sister Claire Maître

Metropolitan Store Explosion, Oct. 25, 1960

PEOPLE WERE SCREAMING. WOMEN WERE SOBBING. THE WALLS HAD COLLAPSED. SLABS OF CONCRETE were strewn about the place, and showers of bricks crushed a half-dozen cars. Small fires had also started throughout the building, as live wires snapped and plummeted into the wreckage. Nineteen-year-old Paul Drouillard, who had been working in the stockroom, clambered through the rubble, accompanied by another employee, Yvette Helwig. The two were searching wildly for a way out. They spotted others picking themselves up from the ground, stunned and shocked by the explosion that had rocked this downtown store. Helwig observed, "There was fire all over. All I could see were bodies buried under rocks and hear children screaming." The two zigzagged their way to rescuers who were rushing to the scene.

This was the Metropolitan Store, a popular dime store, just a few blocks from Hôtel-Dieu Hospital. It was a little after 2 p.m., October 25, 1960. *The Windsor Star* reporter that afternoon described the explosion as "a small earthquake." Indeed. L. J. Arpin of Arpin's Furs was passing a nearby parking lot when he witnessed the conflagration. He said, "I've seen walls go down in my time, but never anything as fast as that. Then the roof closed in on the building like a door. If anyone were in there, they wouldn't have time to think. I saw a man being taken to an ambulance. He told me he had lit the furnace that caused the blast: The ventilating outlet on the roof flew up and down and before it was down, the walls had collapsed. It was two minutes to two by my watch."

People flocked to the debris-ridden main drag of Windsor, in hopes of finding their loved ones alive. "Each time a body was brought out, one could hear sobs, 'Who is it? Who is she? Oh! My God!'" *The Star* reported.

Hôtel-Dieu suddenly launched itself in the "disaster mode" or a set of defined protcols it had only recently introduced. "We were ready," the sisters wrote in their chronicles of that historic and

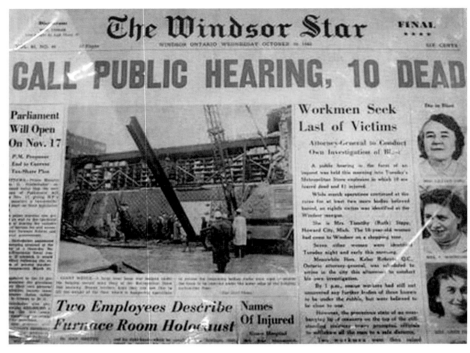

In October, 1960, a gas explosion shook Windsor's Metropolitan Store, killing 10, as reported on the front page of The Windsor Star.

tragic event. A steady flow of ambulances descended upon the facility, and the disaster team was on the phone summoning doctors from all over the city.

Eleven died in the explosion that was triggered by natural gas. The newspaper reported that shards of glass, football helmets, Halloween masks and baldhead mannequins littered the street. Joseph Halford, the 34-year-old manager, was badly burned in the blast, and from his hospital bed, told a *Star* reporter: "I was helping install a new heating unit in the boiler room. We had turned on the gas but nothing came out but air. We then decided, after 15 minutes, to try something else, since no

gas was coming. A plumber's helper got a larger wrench and opened the five-inch valve from the main. More air pushed in and with it must have come gas. We had a small summer heater burning in one corner of the room. I guess when the escaping gas hit that everything went. The roof fell in."

Upwards of a hundred people were rushed to Hôtel-Dieu and Metropolitan Hospital after the blast. *Windsor Star* reporter Walter McCall was among the first to crawl into the building. His article, "I Was In Hell" ran later that afternoon in the paper. He wrote, "For close to two hours I scratched and dug through the macabre world of the 'living and dead." He described his furious search for survivors, and how he helped those who were dazed and shaken, like a little girl "who stumbled through the litter, tears streaming down her soot-covered cheeks."

Dr. John McCabe orchestrated the disaster response at Hôtel-Dieu all afternoon and night. Dr. J. L. Barber assisted. Some 30 victims were hurried to the downtown hospital. The refectory used by the nurses was transformed into a medical ward where victims were attended. Those needing more urgent care were accommodated in regular wards. One man died on the operating table within the first few hours of being brought to Hôtel-Dieu.

"The search for victims went on throughout the night with a lot of bravery from charitable people. In situations like this, there are a lot of caring people, a lot of people with heart.

Many risked their lives to save the victims," wrote the sisters.

At the hospital, teams of nurses, doctors, and the sisters, too, hustled through the night without pausing to go home. The most touching notation in this chronicle was the story of a three-month old baby boy, who three hours after the blast, was found buried in the rubble of the store. He showed a cranial fracture, but finally was diagnosed as being "in good condition" and would be able to go home in a few days. The sisters wrote: "His guardian angel had protected him."

Sister Cecile LeBoeuf

"I didn't want to be a nurse," is what Sister Leboeuf replied when asked about her vocation. "I wanted to be a sister, and I wanted to be a lab technician." But she was a little confused about which order to join. Partly because of her aunts. Two were at St. Mary's Academy, members of the Sisters of the Holy Names of Jesus and Mary. It may be because they were always chatting to her about considering the religious life, and joining them. Another aunt, Laura LeBoeuf, called Sister Marie de la Ferre, at Hôtel-Dieu, whispered nothing to young Cecile. The Holy Names convent had been in Windsor longer, having established itself there in 1864 when Windsor had a population of 3,000. It opened St. Mary's Academy within a month of arriving, and taught at the Catholic Women's College of Assumption in those first 100 years.

Sister Marie de La Ferre simply went about her life saying little about the Religious Hospitallers of St. Joseph. She had also just stepped down from her role as Superior four years earlier when her niece opted to join.

"My aunt never spoke about it—she simply let me decide on my own," recalled Sister LeBoeuf, who added that in a way maybe this was deliberate. "I went to see my aunt once, and she told me, 'I don't think this is for you.' Then she must've felt something because she mentioned it to her Superior, and she said to my aunt, 'Well you should've been more encouraging.' So my aunt invited me to come and visit, and when the decision came to enter, the Religious Hospitallers became my choice."

Much later when Cecile was on a retreat, she was taken aside by Sister Maria de la Ferre: "We were supposed to be silent, but she saw me in a hallway (in the convent) and said to me, 'Now do you think you know what you're doing?' I answered her, 'I always knew what I was doing!'"

From the first day in the convent, Cecile confided to the Superior that she had no intention of working as a nurse; she wanted to be a lab technician. That's precisely what she pursued. Cecile grew up in St. Joachim. She was friendly, hardworking, devoted. Her family had come from Quebec. She was one of eight children. Five became nuns, and a brother, became a priest. The last time she saw him was the night before he died. He had come to Amher-

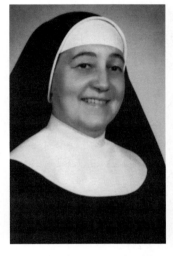

Sister Cecile LeBoeuf, 1965

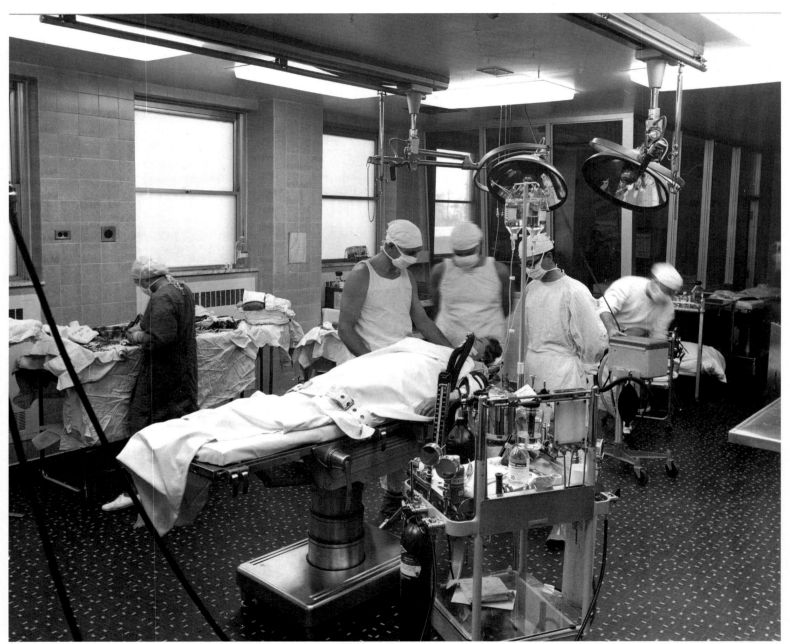

Recovery operating room circa 1965

stburg to give a talk, and she had dinner with him. The next morning, he sat in the church rectory, sipped on a cup of coffee, had a heart attack and died.

As for her vocation, Cecile remarked, "I always felt that if I were a nurse, I'd have so much responsibility, but then I didn't realize what I was getting into until my first day as a (lab) technician. I was on call, and someone whose blood I had checked earlier that day, died. I knew then I really had to put all of my attention on this job. It was greater responsibility than I thought."

When Sister Leboeuf finally entered the convent in 1945, there were 30 nuns living there. Her novitiate was at St. John Evangelist Home for Seniors, which later became Villa Maria, a place that she would later return to as Superior. In 1947, she made her first profession of vows, then continued to St. Mary's Academy. Following this, she enrolled at Assumption to pursue a Bachelor of Science degree. "I was among the only young women taking those courses with pre-meds."

This would lead to a course in medical technology. Later on, she would wind up teaching the students in the lab at Hôtel-Dieu, and serve as its supervisor for 18 years.

"As a lab technician, I was on call every night," she said. "If a patient was sick, I was called. They made us a schedule, but most of the time because I was living in the convent, a step away from the hospital, I was asked to get up. Eventually I became supervisor."

Life in the convent began at dawn, or just before: "We got up for prayers, and then mass, and then prayers again. It was a religious life. Mass was at 6 a.m. Every day."

Sister LeBoeuf continued to pursue courses to broaden her role at Hôtel-Dieu. One was in hospital administration, and it was right after taking this that in 1965 she was named Superior and hospital administrator. She retired from Hôtel-Dieu in 1992, and transferred to Villa Maria to serve as its Superior. In 1997, she celebrated 50 years in religious life. For a brief time, she returned to Hôtel-Dieu to volunteer. Frank Bagatto, Hôtel-Dieu's chief operating officer from 1990 to 2001, said this of Sister LeBoeuf: "She was one of those who would never give up; she had this drive in her. It was there even in her last days here. She was marginalized health wise, but she was out there in the lobby doing fundraising."

Bagatto recognized in this sister something of the way the religious order had operated all those years, how it was maintained, and how its vision for patient care was sincere and faith-based. He believed that sometimes the setbacks made them stronger—even some of the physical impediments like the time Sister LeBoeuf was in the intensive care unit. She had collapsed, and the doctors had predicted it would only be "a few days" before she died. Sister LeBoeuf surprised everyone and survived. In April 2009, she was transferred to St. Joseph Regional House in Amherstview, near Kings-

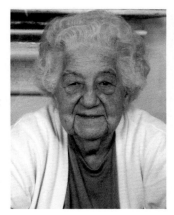

Sister Cecile LeBoeuf

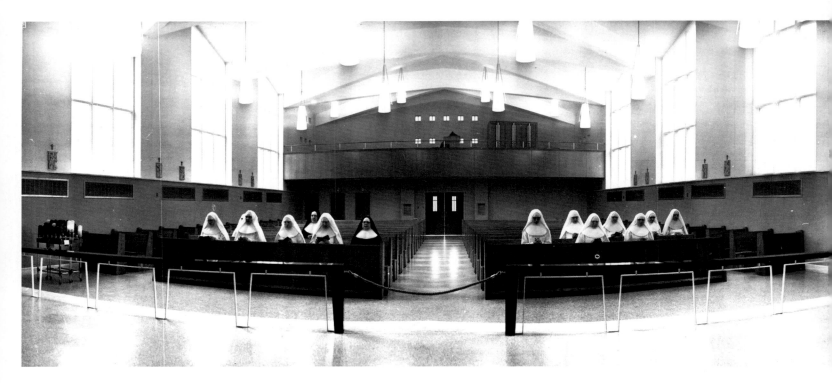

Sisters in the chapel, February, 1964

ton. In September 2012, the majority of the nuns living at this house moved to Heathfield, the Mother House of the Sisters of Providence of St. Vincent de Paul in Kingston.

Roman Mann

Roman Mann's roots with Hôtel-Dieu go back to 1956 when he was hired as an administrative assistant with responsibility over budgets and personnel. When he started there, the hospital had some 800 employees, and he once boasted he knew everybody by their first name. Mann, one of the first lay persons to run a Catholic hospital in Canada, hailed from Saskatch-

ewan. His parents were German-Canadians. They persevered through the Depression years farming and saving every penny they could.

Mann told *The Star* once in an interview that he thought his upbringing helped him to be fiscally responsible. "I think, on balance, being raised then had a good effect on me. I can always look back and see how and what we did…I wouldn't exchange my days as a boy on the farm for anything."

His interest in business lured him to Robertson's Business College in Saskatoon, but not before he obtained a degree in philosophy at a theological seminary. Right out of college,

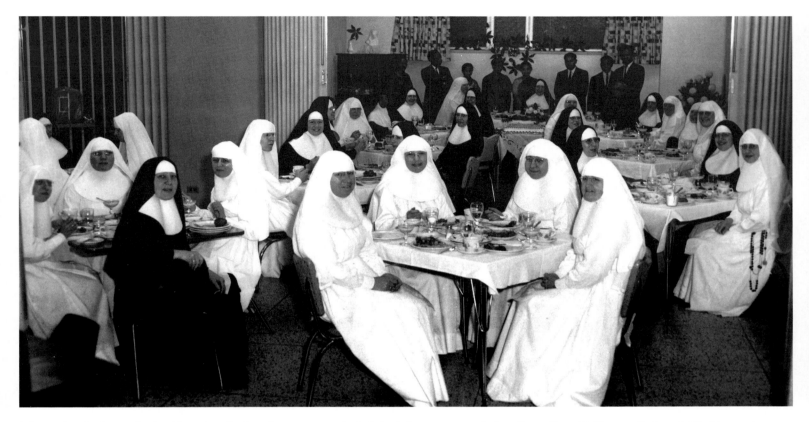

Father J. Chakiamury's annual dinner located in the Hôtel-Dieu cafeteria, 1963

Mann landed a job in Etonia, Saskatchewan where he was secretary-treasurer for the town, hospital and school district. He was also named Justice of the Peace. Mann stayed in Etonia for only three years, but it was long enough to draw him into the health field. In 1954, now married, Mann drove east to take over the administration of Ingersoll Alexandra Memorial Hospital, east of London, Ontario. While there, he also enrolled in courses in Canadian Hospital Management and Organization. He obtained a certificate from the American College of Hos-pital Administrators and the Canadian College of Health Executives.

In 1956, Mann arrived in Windsor and, by 1968, he was Hôtel-Dieu's executive director. In that position, he saw the tear down of the original 1888 structure, and spearheaded the new eight-storey wing. He was also responsible for still more additions and major renovations totaling $25 million at the hospital.

In a 1988 interview with *The Star*, Mann felt "privileged" to have chosen this career: "I think we see the beginning of life and we also

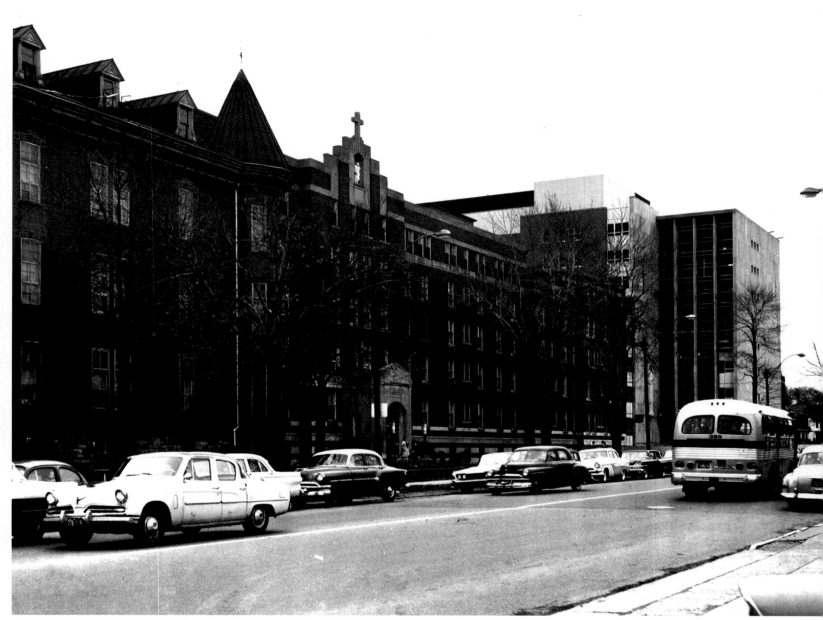

Construction of 1962 wing

see that life when it comes to an end. Hospital people should consider themselves very privileged to be the people instructed to take care of that. It's very special."

Mann was seen as a man with a great sense of humour, and down to earth. He often wandered the corridors to people one on one. He once told a newspaper reporter that the business of running a hospital often is done in the board rooms, when, in fact, this can mean losing touch with the reality of everyday.

The state of health technology and attitudes have also changed dramatically. Mann said, "At one time, you were not required to use extraordinary means to keep people alive. Now the extraordinary has become ordinary. What was heroic in 1956 is very ordinary today."

At the same time, Mann, who succeeded Sister LeBoeuf as administrator, operated with political savvy. A former city hospital authority once commented, "He says and does the right things at the right time. He is a very good chief executive officer as evidenced by the excellent hospital and up-to-date facilities."

Mann stepped down in 1990 after 33 years of working at Hôtel-Dieu. Ronald Marr, then executive director of the Catholic Health Association of Ontario, remarked at his retirement party: "The bottom line, Roman, is you really care. You care for your community, you care for the people who work for you, and you care for the patients in your hospital. For that, all of us thank you."

Frank Bagatto

When he was named chief executive officer of Hôtel-Dieu in 1990, the 47-year-old Italian-born Frank Bagatto probably thought back to his days at the University of Detroit. He had worked at the hospital four summers straight, first as an oxygen porter, and later as an orderly who carted corpses to the hospital morgue.

"I used to tell people I learned the business from the bottom up," Bagatto will say with a laugh. He will also recall those early years, remarking, "It was a different environment when I started there. Nurses looked like nurses; they wore caps, and you knew whether they were registered nurses or graduates, and you admired them. I can remember the doctors, the (Norm) Thiberts and (Clare) Sanborns of the world. They wore ties. And it was also a slower pace then, and people stayed longer. Now it's more of a production medicine."

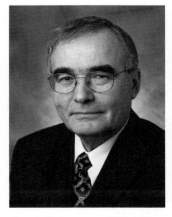

Frank N. Bagatto, Hôtel-Dieu President and CEO from 1990-2002

Bagatto came to Hôtel-Dieu from St. Joseph's Hospital in Sarnia, where he was executive director. In Sarnia, he directed the planning and building of a 200-bed chronic care facility at a cost of $29 million in 1990. He was also the architect of bringing health services in that city under one umbrella. Bagatto had more than 20 years of experience in the health field when he succeeded Roman Mann as CEO. In returning to Windsor, he was coming back to his roots, to the very hospitals whose corridors were as familiar as his home. In essence, Hôtel-Dieu was home.

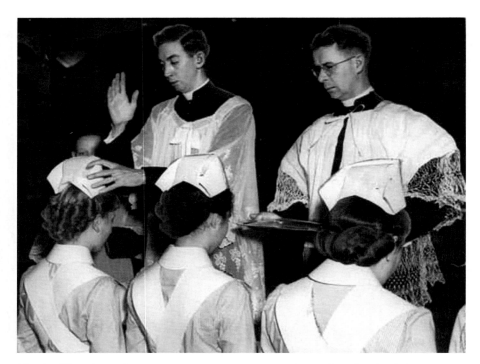

The traditional capping ceremony admitting students to the Hôtel-Dieu School of Nursing was held for 39 students who had successfully completed a four-month preliminary course. In this picture, Violet Braichello is shown as she was capped by Rev. A.L. Meloche. At right is Rev. Pierre Boudreau who assisted.

based commitments is more deliberate than in the past." He said the early days of Hôtel-Dieu saw a significant number of nuns running the hospital and caring for the patients.

Bagatto said, "In one way, they held us accountable, like Sister Gore and Sister Bernadette Gouin, who would roam the corridors and if they saw something in the hallway that needed to be picked up, or something to be fixed, they took care of it. We learned by example, and there were enough sisters in every area of the hospital to have that impact. As the number of sisters changed, we had to be more deliberate of how our mission and values translated into action."

Bagatto said it really didn't matter if the staff was Catholic—it wasn't always Catholic. True enough, even in its earliest days, Hôtel-Dieu hired doctors who were of the Protestant faith. But the attitudes were clear, said the now-retired C.E.O. "But we invite everybody to embrace the values of service to the patient, and that is, treating each person with dignity and respect to our ideas."

Nursing Open to Men

It seems odd today to think this would be an item for the news, but in the summer of 1964, Hôtel-Dieu decided to break tradition and set up a nursing program that would permit men to be trained in its School of Nursing. Four applications were accepted for the Fall term.

Dolly Goldenberg, associate director of

It was in Windsor that he had his greatest impact. First, he brought Hôtel-Dieu and Villa Maria under one board of management, then initiated the dialogue with the Salvation Army which led to the signing of the "Alliance" in December 1993. He was then appointed executive director of Hôtel-Dieu Grace and Villa Maria in April 1994. Bagatto's financial management resulted in surpluses and a sound fiscal future for the hospital.

With respect to the Alliance, Bagatto firmly believed it was a sound choice, but also argued that Hôtel-Dieu didn't lose its grasp on its faith-based roots. "We are still fundamentally the same, but the way we express our faith-the school at the hospital, made the announcement, and also said the hospital had hired Leo Ryan, a male registered nurse as an instructor. He was a native of Toronto, but graduated from the University of Windsor with a diploma in nursing education. Before attending university, he received his nursing training from the Mack Training School for Nurses in St. Catherines General Hospital. At Hôtel-Dieu he was asked to teach pediatrics.

The four male students being admitted were all from Windsor. These students, unlike the female students, were all required to live at home, since there was no accommodation for them at the hospital. Hôtel-Dieu in the past had received applications from men, but these were ignored because it was against the hospital's policy.

The first male nurse to graduate from Hôtel-Dieu was George Boyd, who received his three-year diploma in September 1968. Sixty two nurses graduated that day at a ceremony at the former Cleary Auditorium (now St. Clair College). A photograph of him appeared in *The Windsor Star* showing him with Mrs. Lynn (Patrick) Emmons, the general proficiency award winner and valedictorian and Sister Yvette Hains, the school's director.

When Boyd graduated, the nurses clustered around him, reported *The Star*. George was assigned to work at IODE (The Imperial Order Daughters of the Empire).

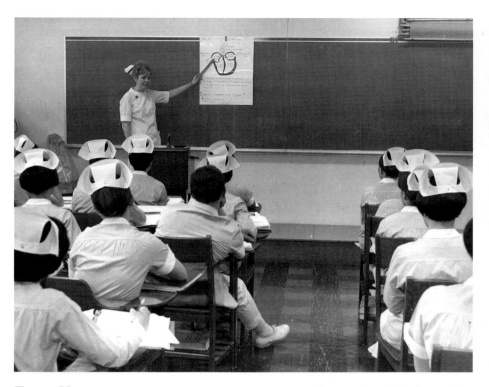

George Boyd, the first male student to graduate, attends class May 8, 1968 at Hôtel-Dieu's School of Nursing.

Expo Nurses

In 1967, Felicia Fanelli was a second-year nursing student at Hôtel-Dieu. The last thing she expected when she signed up for this career was to be running off to Montreal with 96 other nurses to staff the ultra-modern Nurses Station for Intensive Observation at Expo 67. She was accompanied by another nurse, Mrs. Pat Mowat, a supervisor at Metropolitan Hospital.

Fanelli was a good choice since she spoke three languages. She was also voted the school's representative by fellow classmates. Mrs. Mowat was selected by Doris Smith, director of nursing at Metropolitan. The two hospitals

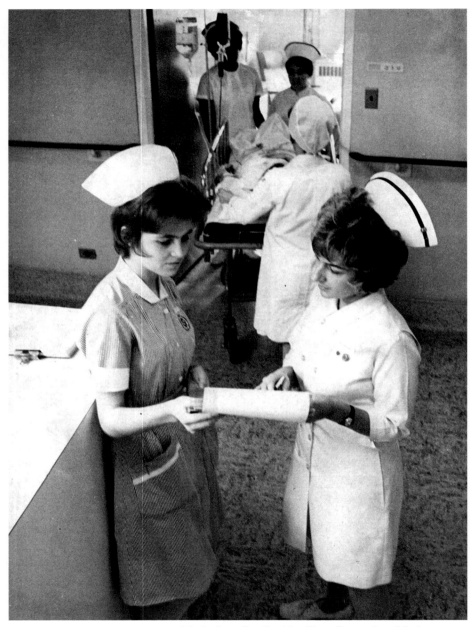

Admission of patient by Floor Supervisor Marie Schiller with student nurse, 1971

were asked to participate by Rita Lussier, coordinator of the project who was assistant director of nursing at Maissoneuve Hospital in Montreal. Fanelli and Mowat were there to demonstrate to visitors at Expo the latest in electronic equipment designed to assist in the care of patients. The nurses chosen for this hailed from all over Canada and the U.S.

The principal exhibit in the nursing station at Expo was a device designed for constant watch on an Intensive Observation unit. This electronic device required a single nurse to sit at a console equipped with television screens. She could then supervise a 10-bed ward.

Inventing Child-proof Prescription Bottle

Dr. Henri Breault

It was Fall 1972 at the Americana Hotel in New York City where a humble, quiet-spoken and earnest man who had grown up in Tecumseh, Ontario, rose to tell a room of doctors and pharmacists that, unless they found a solution, children would continue to be poisoned. He said ramping up the education program—as had been tried in Ontario—did nothing to stem rising numbers of tragic incidents. As a matter of fact, if anything, the figures were soaring higher.

That man—Dr. Henri Breault—then 61 years old, was a pediatrician from Windsor's Hôtel-Dieu, a city and hospital that most at this

New York meeting had never even heard of. Dr. Breault's address to this assembled group of specialists at the American Association of Poison Control Centres was clear. It was passionate. It was direct. It spared no sentiment, except to state that it was about time that real attention was paid to children. In concrete terms, that meant the adoption of a revolutionary child-proof prescription bottle. That's what Breault was selling. He wasn't out to make a buck. That wasn't what anyone was thinking. They knew his passion. He could share tales of rushing through the swinging doors of the hospital to see the limp body of a four-year-old who had swallowed a handful of tiny coloured capsules, thinking they were candies. He could relay to you in meticulous details what it was like to pump the stomach of this child. It was heart breaking. It was tragic. It was wrong.

There were too many instances of this when he would return to his house in Riverside, Ontario, and wonder if there was a better way. That's what motivated him. That's what made the difference.

So, there he was in New York trying to convince the world, beginning first with the poison control specialists. He asked them for "a better approach, something effective, some reliable means of protecting children during the years of greatest risk, those peak years for 95 per cent of all accidental ingestions."

What Breault unveiled that day was the forerunner of today's childproof prescription bottle. It was called "Palm-N-Turn." It had been invented, tested, developed and was now being manufactured in Windsor. Breault and Windsor pharmacist William Wilkinson had dreamed up the world's first such container five years earlier, and turned to International Tools of Windsor for its design and manufacture.

The first hurdle was to convince the Ontario College of Pharmacy. Once they saw Breault's work, their support was enthusiastic. The New York speech, however, was what sent the message to the rest of the world. It proved to be the turning point in convincing North America to follow suit with the poison-control devices.

Breault's daughter, Rosemary Breault-Landry, who eventually went into nursing, recalls those years growing up in that Riverside household. Her father was up and out the door by 6 a.m. "And he was the last one to go to bed at night. He had no cellphone, and we knew his business, and we even answered the phone, and had to be polite, and take messages. People in those days contacted the doctor directly. We had no answering service. We were the answering service."

Rosemary said, "My father went to the hospital every single day, even Christmas, but he was always back in time to open presents, and he was always there for midnight mass." As for the prescription bottles, Rosemary said his passion for developing one that would be childproof started in the late 1950s and early 1960s.

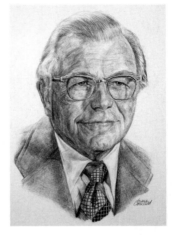

Portrait of Dr. Henri Breault by artist Irma Councill, courtesy of The Canadian Medical Hall of Fame

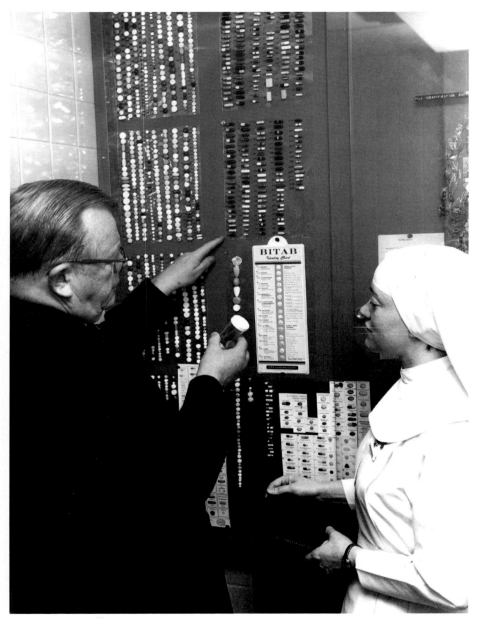

Dr. Henry Breault working with Poison Control, circa 1960

She recalls the "card system" he had devised, and it sat on a table in their house. Those cards would track the occurrences of poison being ingested by children. "My father wanted to know what they were consuming, and sometimes it would be a case where someone had put kerosene into a coke bottle, stored it away, and then the children, thinking it was pop, would consume it." Or, she went on, parents would find their children passed out from having chewed up pills because it was easy to flip open a small plastic container.

"The kids would get up early in the morning, and help themselves, and think it was candy," Rosemary said. That's what led to the establishment of a poison-control centre in Windsor in 1957 at Hôtel-Dieu, the first one of its kind in a hospital. In that first year of its establishment, the centre was dealing with two poisonings per day—800 a year.

As Breault told his New York audience, the centre's first approach—one of education—simply did not work. In an article in *Clinical Toxicology (1974)* he wrote:

> "We went all out. Everyone was educated about the poison hazards in the home. Public, parents, physicians, nurses, mothers, grandmothers, service clubs, P.T.A.s, Home and School organizations, you name it, everyone was alerted and cautioned against the menace..."

The result? In 1966, there were 1,000 poisonings. By 1971, the occurrences of poisonings in Ontario had risen 48% but not in Windsor where the figures seemed to hover at that stagnant number of 800 to 1000 a year. In other words, said Breault, there was little headway being made in the city, but none in the rest of the province.

Meanwhile, the conceptualization continued of a child-proof bottle to put an end to these accidents and to the flood of calls to the poison-control centre where tearful parents turned to the specialists to save their children from dying.

Finally, Breault and his team devised the idea of holding a contest to see if someone could design a child-resistant bottle that might save the lives of children. Rosemary recalls the dining room table covered with these tests.

"My father would test them out on us and other kids. He'd put chiclets in a bottle with some kind of safety cap, and he'd see if we could open them. He also had a lot of older people try them."

The first of these child-proof vials—the Palm-N-Turn, named by Wilkinson and tested at Hôtel-Dieu—convinced Breault and his team that they were "beyond any doubt...entirely effective." More tests were conducted at Huron Lodge among geriatric patients. Half of those used in the study had arthritis,

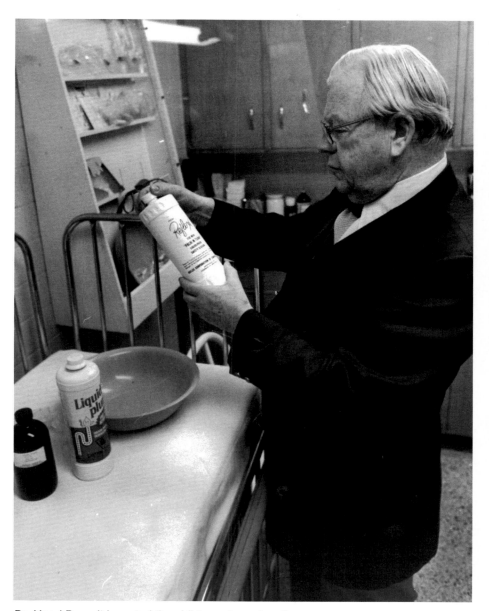

Dr. Henri Breault invented the child-proof cap for pill bottles while working at Hôtel-Dieu. Photo courtesy of The Canadian Medical Hall of Fame.

two were blind, one had Parkinson's Disease, another had cerebral palsy and one had had a stroke with brain injury. Thirty-five patients in all—selected randomly—were chosen, and all but two were unable to pry open the lids. And all had been given specific instructions on how to use them. By January 1967, at the instigation of the Essex County Medical Society and the Essex County Pharmacists' Association, 60 pharmacies in the area were asked to try them in their shops. Five years later, the study proved entirely successful, with a 99-per-cent success rate. Breault was then proud of a chart that he pinned to the wall in the Windsor Poison Control Centre. It displayed all the childhood poisonings in Essex County from all types of products since he started the testing with these new child-proof containers. The graph clearly showed a steady drop from year to year, down 73% in 1972. Meanwhile the graph showed a soaring 48% in the numbers being poisoned in the rest of the province.

Breault and his team delivered hundreds of lectures on their studies, campaigned tirelessly, handed out leaflets, wrote editorials, and appeared on television and radio, to convince the medical world the urgency of the adoption of this new device. Breault, in another speech to Ontario pharmacists, called the incidents of these poisonings "deplorable, a disgraceful situation." He said the medical world had been "entrusted" with the "preservation of God's children," and it was their duty to take the mea-

sures needed to stem the tide on poisonings.

By 1974, provincial legislation was in place, and the Palm-N-Turn was on the shelves of pharmacies in Ontario and other provinces.

In another address—this time to the Canadian Pediatrics Society on the occasion of winning its highest award in 1978—Breault was zealous in his message:

"You just can't keep containers out of their sticky little hands … But what about keeping the contents out of their greedy little mouths?"

Breault's devotion knew no bounds. Rosemary says although her father was prone to making jokes and having fun, when it came to medicine he was another person. So serious. So focused. So caring.

"We were always aware of the research. He'd sit in his little den and write articles on a typewriter. He'd write to Herb Gray or Paul Martin, both of whom were friends. He'd ask them for their help, their support."

When both Rosemary and her sister, Elise, went into nursing, Breault was proud of that decision. He confided in them the best advice. "He wanted us to listen and respect people," Rosemary recounted proudly. "He told us people can't always tell you what's wrong, and so

Hotel Dieu Hits Jackpot of Twins, Five Sets Arrive Within Week

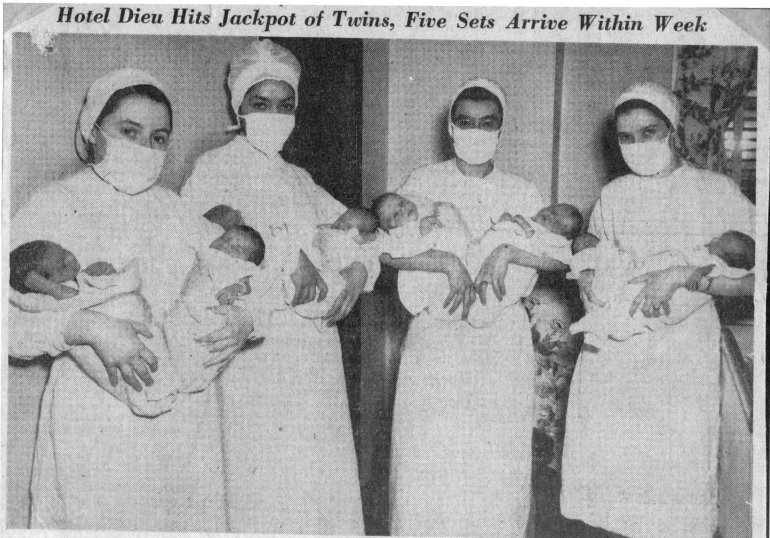

Hotel Dieu hit the jackpot and set a record this week, with five sets of twins in the hospital at once. One set of twins was too tiny to face the camera and remained in the incubator, but the other four make their public debut above in the arms of their nurses. Left to right are Miss Mary Eleanor Walker, holding Paul and Paullette Tracey, children of Mr. and Mrs. Edward Tracey, 405 Eastlawn boulevard, Riverside; Miss Freida M. Parker holding Carol Ann and Carl Fleming, children of Mr. and Mrs. Walter Fleming, 1903 Buckingham drive; Miss Ella H. Bugara, holding Polly and Patricia Quinn, daughters of Mr. and Mrs. Lawrence Quinn, R.R. 4, Essex, and Miss Catherine A. McKeown holding Billy and Beverley Chirko, children of Mr. and Mrs. Joseph Chirko, 672 Partington avenue. (Missing in the picture are Barbara Ann and Beverly Lynn Goyeau, children of Mr. and Mrs. Donald Goyeau, 341 Campbell avenue.)

(Star Staff Photo.)

you always have to listen, and let people explain themselves."

Breault wasn't alive in 1997 for his induction into the Canadian Medical Hall of Fame. As a matter of fact, he was the first physician to be inducted. He joined an illustrious group, including Dr. Frederick Banting and Dr. Charles Best, who discovered insulin. Betsy Little, executive director of the Canadian Medical Hall of Fame at the time of Breault's induction, said, "It's a marvelous, marvelous story because it's so basic and it's someone who persevered and got a problem solved."

Breault's wife, Monica, quoted by Anne Jarvis of *The Windsor Star*, said, "He worked so very, very hard. I'm just sorry he's not around to hear about it." But she recalled the moment of clarity when it all came home. It was 3 a.m., and he was summoned to Hôtel-Dieu to pump the stomach of yet another child. Monica said when her husband returned home, his coat was soiled. He told her, "You know, I've had it. Somebody has to do something about children getting into those pills."

Old Blue Eyes

One of the stories that still circulates around Hôtel-Dieu is the night Mother Marie de la Ferre, the hospital's former Superior, stormed into St Patrick's Ward, thinking Dr. Frank DeMarco, Sr. was up to no good in entertaining the young nurses.

After all, he did have that reputation for being mischievous.

As it turned out, it was a different Frank.

A woman, who had been hurt in an accident, and was now a patient at the hospital, was dismayed that she had to miss a concert in Detroit to hear the legendary Frank Sinatra. A group of friends, feeling sorry for her, managed to convince the crooner to make his way across the river to Windsor and sing for the patient.

The promise was that no one was to know.

Word, however, got out, and about a dozen giggling nurses congregated outside the patient's room to hear Frank Sinatra singing quietly to this patient.

Mother Marie, spotting the nurses assembled there, demanded to know exactly what was going on. The director of nursing quickly told her, 'Not to worry—it is only Frank Sinatra singing for the patient, and he does not want it known that he is there."

To this, Mother Marie responded: "I imagine not!"

PART V

Differing Faiths: One Purpose

1980s-2013

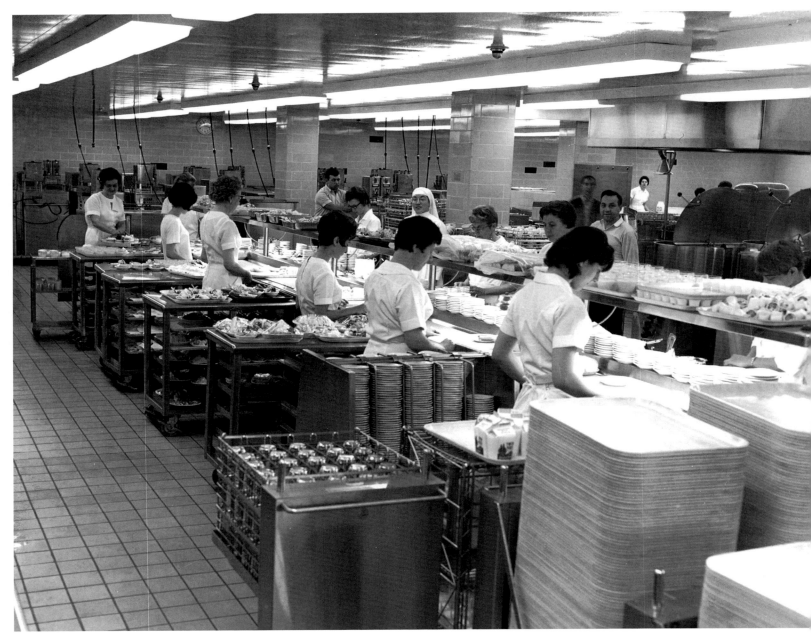

Hôtel-Dieu kitchen, circa 1960s

A Different Tone

THE RELIGIOUS ORDER THAT HAD BEEN RUNNING THE HOSPITAL SINCE 1888 HAD CHANGED DRA-
matically. This was never more evident than when the 1980s approached. It wasn't that the pioneering, work-around-the-clock ethic had disappeared, but the sisters were taking a time out for other activities, other concerns. It did not replace the spiritual. There was no diminishing of devotion or dedication at the hospital; conversion and care of the sick continued unabated. But the nuns were far more relaxed, more in sync with the secular world outside their walls. This would have had Bishop Fallon fuming. In the early days of religious life here, the bishop had complained about the sisters leaving the cloister to go knocking on doors to raise money for the hospital. He worried over their profession. He feared their spiritual life might suffer.

As the nuns entered the late 1970s and early 1980s, the tone had changed. The old concerns may have still been there, but it was different. Scanning the *Annals* for this period, one sees the sisters aging, and the cloistered atmosphere transformed. There were still the regular pastoral visits of the bishops. Both Bishop John Michael Sherlock of London and his Auxiliary Bishop Marcel Gervais continued to stop in, say mass, speak with the sisters, and participate in liturgies, including funerals of the older nuns. But absent were the days of confrontational moments when bishops swept in with arbitrary pronouncements that put the whole community on edge. There was now even a little humour in the way they responded to the bishops. Take the journal notation from January 1981, for example, when Bishop Gervais remarked about their future "survival" as a religious community within Hôtel-Dieu, and stated that unless they went "through crucifixion," their future was in doubt. The sister's sardonic footnote in the *Annals* reads: "We hope that he is not a prophet."

Life was not the same in the late 1970s and early 1980s. The nuns were more open politically and better connected to secular trends than ever before, especially when it came to provincial budgets and how these might affect the hospital. They were also more vocal publicly. For example, in May 1986 the sisters clearly supported some 600 protestors who rallied against the proliferation of strip clubs in Windsor, and demanded a change in the Criminal Code that would outlaw such establishments here.

At the same time, the sisters eagerly celebrated the repatriation of the Constitution. That day—April 17, 1982—the convent sisters hovered around the television to watch the ceremonies with Pierre Trudeau and Queen Elizabeth. They also spent an evening viewing the municipal election results on television when Elizabeth Kishkon was elected as Windsor's new mayor. The nuns wrote in the *Annals*: "The day (November 8, 1982) is filled with sunshine and balmy air, and the voters show up by the thousands...God bless her!"

"...we toasted the newlyweds with fruit cake and champagne."

And who would have thought that the nuns would be rising at dawn—not to pray—but to watch television. On July 29, 1981 the sisters rose to tune into television, and this is what they reported in the *Annals*: "The day of Prince Charles and Lady Diana's wedding. The majority of the sisters got up at the crack of dawn to watch the ceremonies. Most of them had their breakfast in the community room. In the evening, we all watched the re-run of the ceremonies and together we toasted the newlyweds with fruit cake and champagne."

Four days later on August 1, the nuns assembled to watch the film, *The Sinking of the Titanic*.

Reading through the *Annals*, one also notices the sisters more and more making their way out to concerts at the Cleary Auditorium, or visiting the convent's county cottage near Harrow, or driving to LaSalle to pick strawberries, or spending a good long day canning tomatoes in the hospital kitchen. On October 22, 1983, they write: "...making chili-sauce...The aroma attracted others to the kitchen and was a sure sign of Fall; to confirm this, the skies were gray and it rained all day."

There's also the business of the place itself. There was the 1981 election of Sister Cecile LeBoeuf as the new Superior; other sisters travelling to conferences as far away as Chicago; or running off to retreats or the annual art auctions or meeting with the Ladies Auxiliary. There was also the maintenance and expansion of the hospital that continued from one decade to the next. The old concerns of money persisted, and the Ladies Auxiliary was forever coming through with new ways to raise money. In April 1983, the Auxiliary presented the sisters and the hospital board with a cheque of $50,000 for the renovations of the pediatric department. This was big news, but larger still was the announcement the following year (November 30, 1984) when the Ontario Ministry of Health agreed to provide $2.2 million toward renovating the 60-bed unit.

Life was in flux in the 1980s. More renovations to the chronic care department dominated the news in May 1981. Tenders were also opened for the new residence. In August 1981, the grotto was demolished to prepare the way for enlarging the Emergency Department and make a connection from the hospital to the Jeanne Mance Residence. The ground level of the hospital was also being refurbished.

Meanwhile, ever resourceful, the nuns opted to move chronic care patients in September, with the Ministry of Health's approval, to the Viscount Motel next door while the third floor, where they had been housed, was being renovated. The nuns themselves had vacated their own residence years before when it was imperative that they rebuild—and they moved to houses in the neighbourhood.

In 1986, the Ladies Auxiliary was back again, this time with a cheque of $70,000, earmarking the funds for a new ultra-sound unit. The group also promised the hospital that it would up the ante to $100,000 to target the intensive care unit but fundraising, unfortunately, fell short. In April 1987, the Ladies Auxiliary President Rose Vallance presented the hospital with a check of $70,000 for the unit.

Spirituality and belief, however, never disappeared from the convent and hospital. There was a new generation coming up, but the tenderness and care for the spiritual life was still resilient. And still positive in the belief that healing was also God's work. As an example,

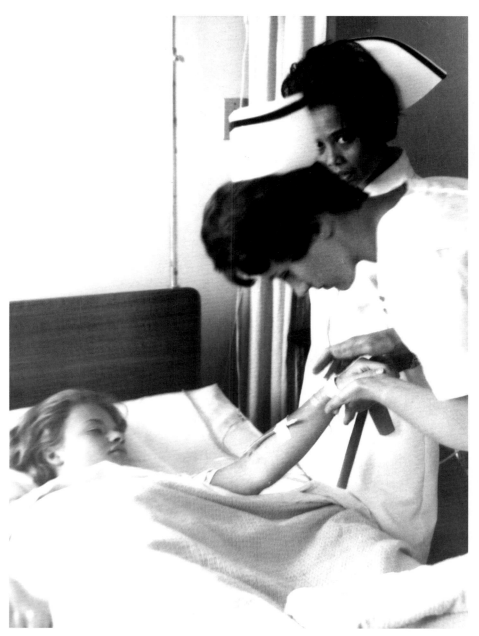

Instructor Patricia Pocock with student nurse, 1969

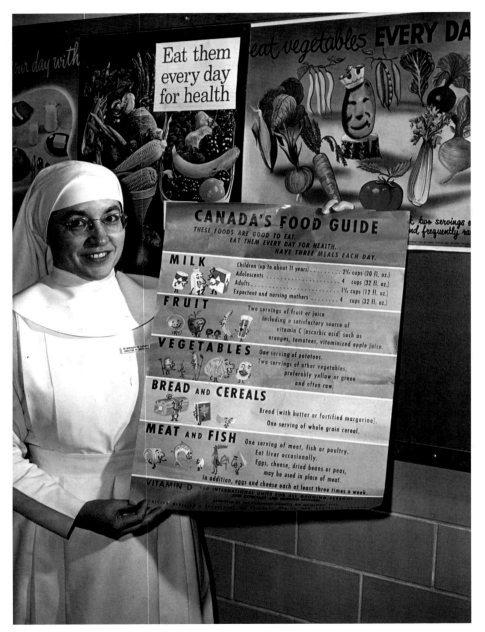

Sister Laporte with the 1965 Canadian Food Guide

Sister Corrona Parenteau, Superior from 1975 to 1981, spoke fondly of a young man who had abandoned the church years ago, suffered a massive heart attack, and one day attended the "healing mass" at the convent chapel. He was "completely healed," wrote Sister Parenteau, and was now entirely devoted to the cause of Hôtel-Dieu. "The other…is a woman who had been given two months to live, and had terminal cancer, and after the Mass as she was prayed over by one of the sisters and a couple of other people, she was completely cured, and after several months, was still fine…"

At the religious order's roots was a genuine compassion for the sick that knew no bounds. In 1990, a St. Catharine's woman involved in a terrible car accident on Highway 401 fractured her clavicle, and was discharged from the hospital, but couldn't drive. Sister Beaulieu quickly offered a room in the convent while arrangements were being made to collect her. The woman had no option, and no place to stay. Such generosity was offered without fanfare.

There was also fierce loyalty to their own. Sister Viola Beaulieu prayed for hours every night at the bedside of Stjepan Hrastovec when he was dying at Villa Maria. He had been Hôtel-Dieu chief of housekeeping for years. His son, Windsor lawyer Peter Hrastovec, said "My father didn't want to be anywhere else. He told me, 'This is a holy place.'"

Also evident in the *Annals*, not just in the 1980s, but throughout these journal-like notations about life at Hôtel-Dieu, was the sincere attention given to those who supported the hospital. The sisters readily acknowledged their debt to such individuals, and when they did, it was couched in the same tone—one of immense gratitude and deep reflection. As an example, on Valentine's Day, 1986, the nuns mourned the death of Mrs. Virginia Fuerth, wife of A. F. Fuerth, former board chair of Hôtel-Dieu, who helped shape the future of the hospital, and who passed away in the late 1970s. The *Annals* also mentioned his grandson Anthony Daniels' ordination in 1983, noting his relationship to Fuerth. Daniels was named auxiliary bishop of London in 2004, and is now bishop of the Diocese of Grand Falls.

In another instance, support for one of their own graduates came in October 1983 when the sisters attended a testimonial dinner honoring Alton Parker of the Windsor Police. Frieda Steele, who was a graduate of the nursing program at Hôtel-Dieu, was Parker's daughter, and she was grateful to see some of the sisters at the dinner honouring her father, the first black detective in Canada. The sisters wrote about him in the *Annals*, saying that Parker was "a very kind and faith-filled citizen."

There were also two individuals from the 1980s that stood out. In May 1983, the sisters spoke affectionately about the legendary Basilian priest, Father Stan Murphy, who had been under their care for many months. He died the evening of May 22. Murphy was the founder of the Christian Culture Series at Assumption, and the one responsible for hiring media icon Marshal McLuhan and artist and writer Wyndham Lewis to teach at Assumption, or the future University of Windsor. The second individual was Dr. Breault, the celebrated pediatrician. He died September 5, 1983. He was retired, but had continued to dabble in work, especially with the child-proof prescription bottles he had pioneered. His contribution at Hôtel-Dieu was revolutionary, and a testament to the way the hospital was governed under their tutelage.

Four Days in September 1984— a Pope, a Birth and a new Prime Minister

It was September 13, 1984. Feast of the Exultation of the Holy Cross. This was the anniversary of the arrival of their Mother Foundress and her companions from Montréal who started this hospital in Windsor, the first in the area. The sisters wrote in the *Annals: We remember this day with grateful hearts, and ask our blessed Lord to continue to bless us as we render service to the sick of our city."

But the day was special in another way. Nine sisters from Hôtel-Dieu—Sisters LeBoeuf, Garceau, Piche, Laframboise, Emery, Bondy, Bachand, Laporte, Adeline—were off to Downsview, Ontario to see Pope John Paul II, who was on a cross-Canada tour. The sisters would join a crowd of 500,000 at the airport near Toronto. They wrote: "Weather condi-

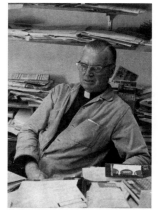

Father Stan Murphy was a Basilian priest at Assumption University in Windsor.

tions were not the best, but no one became ill from the exposure." The night before, there had been a steady rain on the field where the Pope was to celebrate mass. The wind was also brisk and cold. The inclement weather improved by 9 a.m. but the day was cloudy with infrequent sunny periods. As the *Annals* reported: "Hopes and excitement ran high seeing our Holy Father… What joy with the helicopter arrived— flanked by four other helicopters. From the air over the gathered throngs, our white-clad Pontiff waved and greeted the people below… A lasting memory! Thanks be to God!"

The sisters returned home that night:

> "For many, meant hours of travel— but, oh, so worthwhile. In the early hours of Sunday morning, when we arrived in the convent, we found that the sisters who had stayed home, did foresee the fatigue of the travelers, and hot soup and beverages were awaiting us in the kitchen. God bless them!"

It was at that point, in turning on the news, they discovered that Princess Diana had given birth to a son. Three days later, on Sept. 17, Brian Mulroney was sworn in at Government House as Canada's newest Prime Minister.

New Pediatrics Wing

At a special board meeting September 27, 1984, tenders for the Renovation Program of the Pediatric Unit were opened. Adine Construction was awarded the $1.7 million contract. The work would be done in two phases, to be completed by 1986. The sisters noted in their *Annals* that the hospital costs were dramatically different in the 1980s from what they were in the 1880s. In 1888, the nuns charged one dollar per day for a hospital bed. One hundred years later, the all-inclusive daily rate for an in-patient at Hôtel-Dieu was $300.

A New Year, A New TV

New Year's Day 1987 was a mild day for several sisters visiting their families. Others stayed home to watch a videotape of the movie *Amadeus, the life of Mozart*. Sister LeBoeuf brought the tape home from her niece at Christmas. The sisters had to watch it on a borrowed television. Their own had broken down on New Year's Eve. Before watching the film, Mother LeBoeuf drew up a report of the hospital statistics for 1986. Hôtel-Dieu recorded 12,653 in-patients, and 121,033 out-patients. A stellar year.

The next morning the nuns awoke to snow on the ground, the first snow of the year that stayed. That evening the sisters watched another video, "Anne of Green Gables." Three days later, on Jan. 5, the sisters went shopping for a new TV. They picked up an RCA with a stand for the VCR and storage for cassettes. The TV came in handy in October 1987 when the nuns gathered to watch the Detroit Tigers snatch the

"The next morning the nuns awoke to snow on the ground…and went shopping for a new TV…"

American League East Division Championship from the Toronto Blue Jays.

No thanks!

Exotic dancers from Windsor's strip clubs were taken aback when Hôtel-Dieu turned down a donation in February 1987. Auxiliary Bishop Frederick Henry supported the hospital's position. The board also agreed with the decision to inform the strippers their money was not welcome. Roman Mann, Executive Director of the hospital, told the board he was not aware that any of the local charitable institutions or hospitals had accepted the donation. The *Windsor Star*, however, reported that the Salvation Army had decided to accept the donation. The hospital's decision, of course, was in keeping with the sisters' earlier endorsement of a proposal for an amendment to the Criminal Code to ban strip clubs altogether.

Long Time Friend

At the end of June 1987, the sisters learned of the death of Irene Page. She was a long-time friend and major benefactor of the hospital. The sisters praised her accomplishments and great generosity. Page had spent most of the Second World War helping to find homes for displaced children in Europe. She also worked with the United Nations Relief and Rehabilitation Association from 1945 to 1947. She was a child welfare specialist in the Hanover region in Germany. Page joined the International Ref-

ugee Organization as chief counseling officer in Indiana, and later as a child welfare officer in Italy. She had served as a social services officer with the Royal Canadian Army Medical Corps. In the 1960s, Page was appointed as Director of Mental Health Services at St. Thomas Psychiatric Hospital. From 1950 to 1956, she taught sociology at Assumption University. She was also secretary at the Windsor branch of the Red Cross Society from 1950 to 1951. As well, Page was the assistant superintendent of the Roman Catholic Children's Aid Society. The sisters wrote: "We feel very proud of this woman who demonstrated such feelings for her fellow-man and who did not hesitate to bring her many talents to fruition. May she be rewarded for her undaunted courage and generosity in the service of our dear Lord."

Page's funeral was held at St. Rose Parish. Sisters LeBoeuf, Garceau, Noel, Bachand and Laframboise attended.

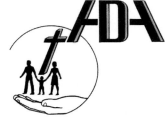

The 1987 prize-winning logo designed by Pina Perichelli for Hôtel-Dieu Hospital

A Logo for Hôtel-Dieu

Employees of the hospital were invited to design and produce a logo for ongoing use by Hôtel-Dieu. On July 23, 1987, the selection committee announced the winner, selected from 23 submissions. Pina Perichelli, a transcriptionist in the Medical Records Department, had the winning design, a hand reaching out to a family (three figures) with the cross above it. The prize was a round-trip ticket for two, either to Toronto, Ottawa, Montréal or

Washington DC. A second-place prize was awarded to Celia Bell, a technician working in the radiology department. As well, each entrant received $25.

Fire

New furniture for the renovations of the hospital, as well as some used furniture and equipment, was destroyed November 21, 1987 in a multimillion-dollar blaze in an aging warehouse. The convent's *Annals* described how "huge fireballs …and hissing flames" shot into the night air Saturday evening. This building contained several other businesses as well as the storage space rented by Hôtel-Dieu Hospital. All the contents in a storage unit were destroyed. Investigators suspected an arsonist, because the fire broke out in about four different areas of the warehouse. One hundred barrels of assorted solvents, and a huge inventory of corrugated paper fed the raging inferno. Damage was estimated at $7 million.

Centennial

When The Religious Hospitallers of St. Joseph in Windsor celebrated their 100th anniversary, 75 sisters came from different houses across the world. Ten were housed at the convent, while the others were accommodated at Holy Redeemer College. The celebration started on May 18 with a mass at St. Alphonsus church. There was a spectacular scene in the church, a very emotional moment at the offer-

"…a dozen red roses in memory of the deceased nuns who served in Windsor."

tory when Sister Evelyn Emery carried a dozen red roses in memory of the deceased nuns who served in Windsor. The flowers were donated by the Hôtel-Dieu Hospital Auxiliaries.

After the mass, the Centennial Parade, numbering 700, left from the church to walk to Hôtel-Dieu Hospital. The parade was led by a police escort on motorcycles followed by a police car with the Chief of Police, John Hughes, and his wife Leona, a graduate nurse of Hôtel-Dieu. A Centennial banquet took place at the Cleary Auditorium that evening.

For Someone Special

It was Thanksgiving Day, 1989. Mass was held in the chapel for the repose of the soul of David Jaggs, who was killed in a motorcycle accident in California where he lived with his wife, Janine. His father, Ken Jaggs, was an Anglican clergyman, and lectured widely. He was in Toronto at the time of the accident. Jaggs was well known for speaking out on drug and alcohol problems. His son's death was a result of the misuse of both. The Sisters of the Religious Hospitallers of St. Joseph in Windsor had enormous respect for Jaggs, and despite his Protestant background, consented to the mass in honor of his son. This Anglican minister possessed strong leanings to the Catholic faith. The journals of the nuns reveal how much affection he had fostered with this faith-based hospital and its Catholic administrators. The saddened family used the moment of the funeral to put greater stress on the dangers of alcohol and drug abuse. David's brother, Andrew, addressed his companions in high school, and underlined the damage done by drug and alcohol abuse. In the hospital journals, we read about Reverend Jaggs' belief that his son David was now in Heaven. "This is where different faiths have a common meeting ground," the sisters said.

Three-Alarm Fire

The nuns at Hôtel-Dieu were watching the news on November 21, 1989, and witnessing the fall of the historic 37-mile-long Berlin Wall. They saw thousands of East and West Berliners streaming to see this five-metre-high wall crumble. Cars were bumper-to-bumper for 12 miles, and Berliners on both sides chiseled at the concrete structure. That same day, at Hôtel-Dieu a welding crew, in the process of boring an 8-inch pipe in an abandoned metal shaft on the third floor, caused a major fire. The nuns recount this in their journals: "Sparks from the torch ignited the insulation around this pipe. Flames shot straight up to the eighth floor. The chute was like a giant chimney belching with fire and smoke." Damage on the third, sixth and seventh floors was estimated at $500,000. The hospital was forced to evacuate the psychiatric patients on the eighth floor. Some were sent home; others were dispatched to local hospitals. The surgery department was shut down due to smoke contamination. The

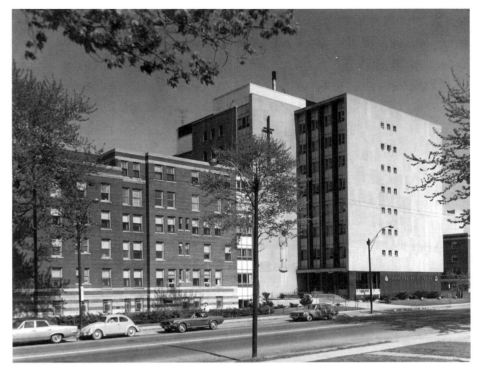

May 8, 1968, entrance on the West side

Fire Chief praised the hospital for its "splendid prompt execution of the hospital fire plan." He said that the emergency systems were well organized. The last fire drill had actually taken place two weeks earlier. Hôtel-Dieu staff in the midst of this fire had sealed off the fire zone, moved quickly to their appointed stations, and transferred patients at risk to the cafeteria in the basement. The hospital was forced to put special crews into action to work around the clock to cleanse equipment in the operating rooms. Only special critical cases were dealt with over the next few days.

New Blood

Fall of 1989 brought new blood to Hôtel-Dieu. Villa Maria, gradually becoming part of the hospital's administration, hired a part-time financial development officer, Luann Kapasi, as well as the new Chief Executive Director, Frank Bagatto, who on April 21 told the media that the key to a Christian hospital in the Catholic tradition was to live the ideal that Christ set for them. That meant in real terms serving those in need, with a greater emphasis on the individual. He stressed that the sisters were still "in control of the operation." Bagatto saw his role as administrator as running the hospital "according to their (the sisters') ideal." This was heartening for the sisters to read in the *Windsor Star*.

As a sign that life still functioned the same way, four days later the Ladies Auxiliary handed over a cheque for $90,000 to Hôtel-Dieu. The Auxiliary also pointed out to the new administrator that they had contributed a total of 29,358 hours of volunteer work, time donated by 198 active members, including 14 men and 40 high school students.

One of Bagatto's first actions was to merge Villa Maria and Hôtel-Dieu. Both were already under the auspices of the Religious Hospitallers of St. Joseph, but the new hospital administrator in May 1990 sought a way to integrate both facilities in a beneficial way. From the point of view of the patient, he said, the hospital could provide tremendous benefits, care and service with the union, especially in the area of support service, education and mission.

The next big move was acquiring more hospital property. After months of negotiations, Hôtel-Dieu snatched up the former Viscount Hotel parcel of land for $4.2 million to accommodate the hospital's need to develop and expand ambulatory services, outpatient clinics, day services, and parking facilities.

Roman Mann officially stepped down as administrator in February 1990. Some 500 guests turned out to his retirement party at the Caboto Club to pay tribute to his three decades of service at Hôtel-Dieu. Sister Beaulieu, now Superior, said Mann's contributions to the hospital had been great, citing the introduction of new medical technologies and expanded programs for the hospital and community. Mann spoke about his 33 years at Hôtel-Dieu. He said the pivitol goal for him was always to keep the focus on the needs of the patient. In the journals written by the nuns, Mann was described as "a true leader."

Reaffirming Its Future: The Alliance

In January 1992, immediately following New Year's Eve, Hôtel-Dieu signed a Declaration of Intent with Grace Hospital to explore options for collaboration so the services provided to the community could be maintained and enhanced. The sisters stressed in their chronicles: "This is an innovative historic first step with many unknowns but motivated by a desire to service, consistent with our Mission and Values."

Sister LeBoeuf and Bagatto left for Montreal that January to attend the provincial Council meeting, during which time the two would explain the *Declaration of Intent* to the provincial and general councils of the Religious Hospitallers of St. Joseph. This agreement arose out of a major discussion paper called "Vision for the Future." It concluded that the continued operation of Windsor's four hospitals would not be in the best interest of the whole community, and would lead to "a steady deterioration of services."

Eight months later, in September 1992, Sister Therese Robert, Provincial Superior, met with the 18 remaining sisters at the Hôtel-Dieu convent. The purpose was to speak to them about their future, and assist them in reaffirming their purpose. Of the 18 still in the convent, the majority were already retired. Some had continued to volunteer at Hôtel-Dieu and five still worked full-time in the hospital. According to the *Annals*, the sisters, indeed, were apprehensive over the future of their order, and their life in the hospital setting. Behind them was a very rich history—a story abundant in mission and purpose. With no new postulants, the hospital's sisters had been forced many years ago to reach beyond their own cloistered walls to find lay people to fill the jobs they once had. Windsor's situation was not unique, Sister Robert said. "The sisters are very well aware of the current events," she explained, "They are very supportive by their interest and by their prayers, especially the rights of the patients and of the population at large, to safeguard the Catholic character of the hospital."

On September 10, 1992, Hôtel-Dieu issued an ominous press release with regard to this future:

> "What concerns the sisters is the several factors which must be excluded—*Religious Affiliation*: Multi-denominational pastoral services must continue to be assured at all facilities, but beyond that, religious affiliation will not be considered in the assessment; *Governance*: the government structure must serve the needs of the system; *Management Performance*: Therefore, current management performance is not an important factor in predicting future management performance within any new configuration."

Nearly two years later, the years ahead that Sister Robert alluded to now was becoming a reality. In February 1994, the media's attention focused on major changes to city hospitals. Two hospital boards were established to oversee the combined operations at Windsor Western and Metropolitan hospitals and Hôtel-Dieu and Grace. As the newspaper pointed out, the steering committee's ambitious plans could not be

"Behind them was a very rich history— a story abundant in mission and purpose."

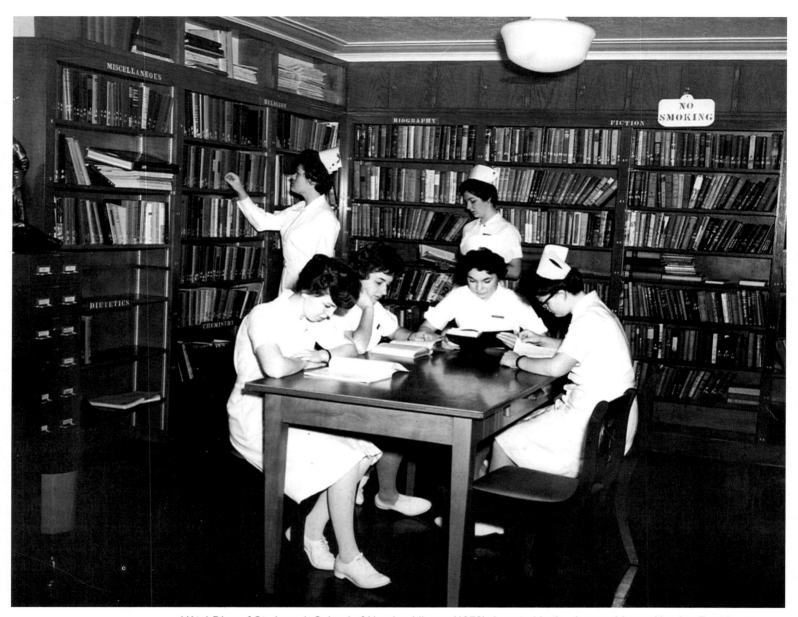

Hôtel-Dieu of St. Joseph School of Nursing Library (1973). Located in the Jeanne Mance Nursing Residence (1946 Building), which was closed in 1975. Not to be confused with the Medical Library (formerly Doctor's Library) that was still located in the hospital (1962 wing).

given the green light until approval came from the Ontario Ministry of Health. The anxiety is evident in the jottings in the chronicles of the nuns: "We still need to pray with faith and hope."

Reconfiguration

Through the early part of the 1990s, Hôtel-Dieu arranged a series of Town Hall meetings to address questions about the process of reconfiguration regarding the alliance with Grace. The staff in these sessions never held back; neither did the Catholic hospital's CEO. Bagatto maintained it was imperative to explain the process, and how the scope and funding of the services should be improved in the community by this alliance. Meanwhile, summits between the Salvation Army Territorial Head Quarters Governing Council and the sisters were scheduled, so that a contract could be prepared with input from both owners. Sister Rose Marie Dufault of Hôtel-Dieu did her best in tackling the issues that affected future patients as a result of this proposed alliance. She voiced the pending agreement and its implications on French radio in November 1993. A month later, it became clear that if the alliance were to work, it would necessitate a genuine sharing and willingness to cooperate. The symbolic gesture of this took place December 4, 1993 when, for the first time, the staff at Grace and Hôtel-Dieu celebrated Christmas together at the Caboto Club. More than 600 attended. The night was magical—it was marked by an impressive candlelight ceremony to announce the formal alliance between the two hospitals.

Four days later, Hôtel-Dieu's Bagatto and Lt. Col. Docheray of the Salvation Army held yet another Town Hall meeting, this time inviting the staff of both hospitals to celebrate this "historical moment." On December 9, 1993, a press conference was convened in the Hôtel-Dieu Hospital auditorium, and a ceremonial signing took place. Hospital authorities agreed that their expectation was that both hospitals would move quickly to operate as one corporate entity by April 1, 1994. The sisters penned in their *Annals* that this merger was "the first such agreement of this scope ever signed in Canada." The press conference drew more than 300 people, mostly medical staff. At the ceremonial signing, representatives of both hospitals lit a white candle with two wicks to symbolize the alliance.

In an effort to include all employees in the formal event, Grace Hospital rented a Transit Windsor bus to shuttle employees back and forth to Hôtel-Dieu every half hour. Hôtel-Dieu itself was festooned with Christmas decorations, and the hospital arranged high tea to be served with sterling silver and china by the sisters themselves. The chroniclers in the *Annals* wrote that the day was one of high emotions: "There were a few tears shed, knowing that Hôtel-Dieu of St. Joseph in Windsor will never be the same."

"The night was magical…marked by a…candlelight ceremony to announce the formal alliance…"

Looking at The Future

The sisters gathered on the weekend of September 15, 1995 for a historic retreat led by Sister Kathleen Lichti of the Adult Spirituality Center of Windsor. She was a member of the Sisters of St. Joseph of London, and well known as a leadership facilitator. Sister Kathleen was also a former Superior and administrator for a religious order. The retreat opened Saturday morning at 9 a.m. with the goal of examining the future needs of the religious community and its place in Windsor, but more specifically as part of Hôtel-Dieu.

According to the *Annals*, the day was spent "in remembering, sharing and rediscovering (their) roots, values, strengths, and (their) reality…for an aging community, and an uncertain future in its present home." Tensions were high. The workshop was held on Sunday morning, and the sisters were asked to brainstorm options for the future. By the afternoon, two participants dropped out, and one refused to participate.

The workshops continued until October. On Sunday, October 1, 1995, a warm day, Sister Kathleen held the final session. Several nuns were still divided over what the future would bring. In the *Annals*, the sisters wrote: "Was this workshop to be helpful?" The answer, according to the convent's report was:

"At this time it seemed not, but it did serve to awaken us to the fact that the

"There were a few tears shed, knowing Hôtel-Dieu of St. Joseph will never be the same."

change was imminent, and whether we accept it or not, it will happen."

Two days later, on October 3, it was official. The name of the front of the hospital in the lighted display now read "Hôtel-Dieu Grace Hospital." The old familiar sign "Hôtel-Dieu of St. Joseph" was gone. As the sisters will tell you, this caused great pain for many of the senior nuns. It certainly was coincidental that, over the next few days, the convent experienced some bizarre occurrences. Thanksgiving weekend it rained so hard that the east-facing windows on the fourth floor of the convent, though closed, could not keep the water out. Sister Bondy kept mopping up the deluge. She placed mounds of flannel blankets on the floor to soak up the rainwater. A few days later, at the front of the hospital where the city was repairing Ouellette Avenue, Sister Garceau and Sister Piche, both then in their late 80s, stumbled and fell in the middle of traffic. They were nearly run over by motorists. A gentleman got out of his car to assist them across the street safely. He made sure they were able to manage on their own. Both sisters suffered scrapes and were taken care of in emergency. They also promised to no longer go out on their own.

The Reality

The merger with Grace Hospital was far from easy. On February 20, 1996, a Town Hall meeting was held in the auditorium at Hôtel-

Dieu regarding the signing of a partnership of Hôtel-Dieu Grace, the Windsor Regional Hospital, the Leamington District Memorial Hospital and the District Health Council. A few days earlier, Armando Deluca, board chairman of Hôtel-Dieu Grace Hospital Board of Directors held an open forum in the auditorium at King Edward Public School. The goal was to give the public an opportunity to present issues and concerns regarding the changes at Hôtel-Dieu and Grace. Questions were raised over the viability of the kidney dialysis unit at Grace. Some also worried over the closing of Chronic Care at Hôtel-Dieu. Chronic Care patients were scheduled for transfer to Grace, a move that had been anticipated when the merger was presented. Indeed, this relocation took place on March 5. It particularly upset Sister Regina Piche who, at age 89, was still working with the chronically ill, visiting them three days a week. As the chroniclers state in the *Annals*, "She spoke with them, prayed, consoled and comforted them."

By April 1996, the Emergency Room at Grace was closed; the staff that worked there were relocated. Bagatto, meanwhile, maintained his positive attitude for the alliance of the two hospitals, and reminded the staff that negative stances would reflect upon patient care. He held another Town Hall meeting in October 1996 to review the process Hôtel-Dieu had been through with the alliance with the Salvation Army Hospital. The sisters felt the open forum gave the staff the opportunity to vent their frustrations.

Grace Hospital

Grace Hospital came into being somewhat the same way as Hôtel-Dieu. It was out of a need in the community. Politicians and medical authorities were all of one mind: there was a pressing need for more hospital beds in Windsor. Hôtel-Dieu could never function independently, especially in an environment where the city was beginning to boom with an auto industry in the early stages of transforming society. The Salvation Army listened to those needs in those early years of the 20th century. It finally, stepped forward and purchased the former Ellis home at Crawford and London Street. The idea from the start was to open it as a maternity hospital since that had been the tradition of the Salvation Army in other parts of the country. The pressing community need, however, was for a facility that could take the overflow from Hôtel-Dieu. Naturally, there were the detractors, who thought a "Catholic" hospital ought to be a more "general" facility.

Initially, the new facility opened in 1918 with 28 beds. The strain of an influenza epidemic tested its facilities. This fueled the decision for expansion. In 1922 a new wing was added, thereby providing more than a hundred additional beds. It wasn't until 1942 that a new South Wing was opened, adding another 80 beds. This also included a new pediatrics ward,

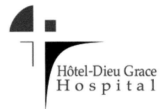

A new logo was designed for the new Hôtel-Dieu Grace Hospital.

Album of Grace Hospital Graduates

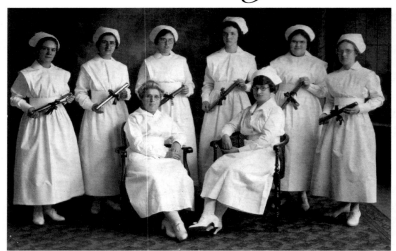

Grace Hospital graduating class of 1924

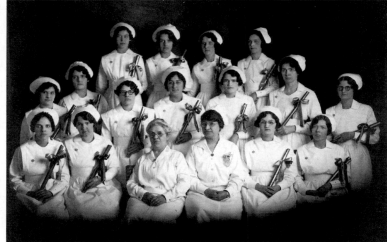

Grace Hospital graduating class of 1929

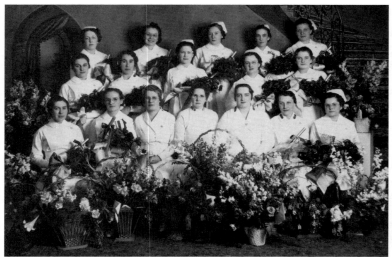

Grace Hospital graduating class of 1939

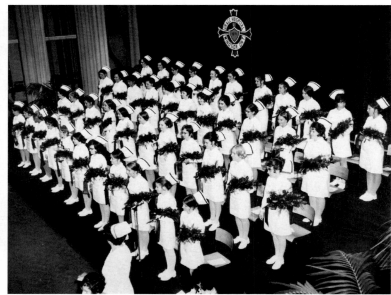

Grace Hospital graduating class of 1971

classrooms and a library. To accommodate the nursing training, Grace bought five nearby residences to house its students until it could provide a Nurses' Residence in 1954.

Grace's School of Nursing operated for 53 years from 1920 to 1973 and graduated 1,529 nurses.

More construction was needed in 1945, with administrators adding a north wing. In June 1960, fire ripped through the oldest part of the hospital, necessitating further construction. A new five-storey wing with air conditioning officially opened in September 1966. The original structure was all but gone except for the central door of the Ellis home. This was showcased in the main lobby area of the 1966 wing. That door is now lcated next to Emergency and Admitting on Goyeau Street.

Windsor fell under the orders of the Provincial Ministry of Health to save money by eliminating a duplication of services. Grace Hospital reacted to this in 1972 by setting up an 'In Common Laboratory'. It also shut down its pediatric department. In 1979, it established a 25-bed Chronic Care Unit in its North Wing, and two years later opened an ultramodern Cardiac Care Unit. In February 1980, the hospital went ahead with its new West Wing, and added 54,000 square feet to its Perinatal Unit, Emergency, Rehabilitation, Respiratory Therapy and Materials Management Departments. The West Wing was officially opened in March 1985.

The changes that led to the eventual demo-lition of Grace began with the Alliance Agreement in mid-1991 when the Chief Executive Officers from both Hôtel-Dieu and Grace started discussions of the advantages of sharing services.

In December 1993, after two years of planning, the Alliance Agreement was signed and went into effect on April 1, 1994. It actually brought three facilities—Grace Hospital, Hôtel-Dieu and Villa Maria Home For the Aged—under one corporate structure. Soon, this led to one site—Hôtel-Dieu Grace on Ouellette Avenue. The Grace site was closed February 1, 2004 and demolished in the Spring of 2013. Villa Maria was closed as a long term care facility. Its building and land were transferred to the University of Windsor.

Through architect Orien Duda's initiative and Bill Marra, the Hôtel-Dieu Foundation's president, the Grace Hospital and Grace Nursing Residence cornerstones were saved from demolition and given to Hôtel-Dieu Grace Archives.

Funding

March 12, 1996 was a good news day for Hôtel-Dieu. Frank Bagatto, the hospital's chief executive officer, was all smiles when he strolled into Sister Bernice Bondy's office. He told her capital funding for the restructuring of the hospital had now been approved by the provincial government. Finally, Hôtel-Dieu was able to complete the reconfiguration process that had

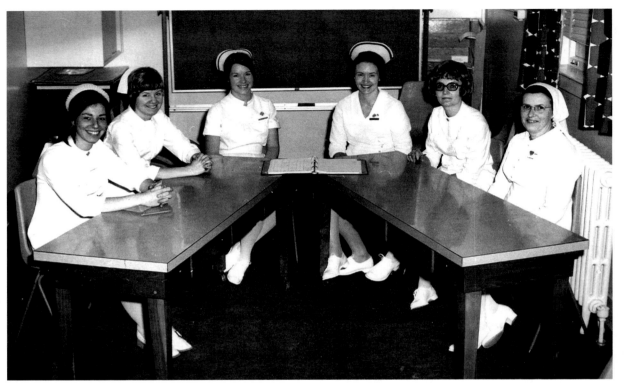

Medical Surgery teachers in 1971, (left to right) Miss. Venable, Mrs. Stuart, Mrs. Gregor, Mrs. Pocock, Mrs. Surgent, Sr. Lajeuneusse

begun several years and two governments ago. It was Bob Rae's New Democratic government that had given the green light to this major building project, but Mike Harris' Conservative Government had postponed the funding.

The good news didn't last long. Almost a year later, on January 29, 1997, Bagatto fired harsh words at the Ontario government in a scathing open letter that accused the province of severely "underfunding" Windsor's health care. He pointed out that the provincial average was $718 million, whereas Windsor's was $596 million, a $42 million shortfall. Meanwhile, he said, the city's hospitals were stretched to the limit, and that patients were being discharged too early to make room for others. Bagatto also said those needing critical care were being placed in other units, and elective surgeries were being cancelled.

The Windsor Star described Bagatto's letter as "blowing the whistle" on the provincial Tories. Its editorial writers argued that for nearly 10 years, Essex County had been "knee deep in health care reconfiguration," and that three successive governments had praised this community "for putting turf wars aside to come up with innovative ideas that will save money and lives."

Windsor, to its credit, had managed by 1997 to turn four hospitals into two, and was still struggling to slash more in spending, while the rest of Ontario was enjoying the benefits of higher funding. Windsor had been "played the fool," and had been "cheated," concluded *The Star*.

Bagatto, that day, was a hero to Essex County, but his voice didn't change the health-care landscape immediately. The hospitals in Windsor continued to be overcrowded, and its emergency rooms were mired in chaos.

Meanwhile on that day that Bagatto's letter appeared, the nuns were gathered gleefully around a new refrigerator that had just been delivered to the convent. They were surprised that their CEO, a man known for diplomacy, had penned such a scathing open letter calling the provincial government into question. But they also knew it had to be voiced.

The Office of the CEO

Neil McEvoy

Neil McEvoy was hired as the CEO for Hôtel-Dieu Grace in 2004, and departed the hospital in September 2008. He came to Windsor from Kingston, Ontario where he had served as the Associate Executive Director at that city's Hôtel-Dieu. He brought some 16 years in the health field to the job in Windsor. McEvoy was described by Sister Rosemarie Kugel, president of the Religious Hospitallers of Hôtel-Dieu of St. Joseph, as "an energetic champion of individual development and effective teamwork among staff."

Bill Marra, past board chairman, and now president and executive director of Hôtel-Dieu Grace Foundation, said McEvoy "should be proud" of his work in Windsor. For one, despite the controversy that surrounded the hospital, he managed to bring into being initiatives that led to four consecutive surplus budgets in tough economic times.

Warren Chant

Warren Chant was hired in June 2009 as the CEO. He had been CEO at Leamington District Memorial Hospital for 13 years. When Ken Deane was appointed by the province as supervisor, Chant was forced to leave. "While I am disappointed," he said, "I respect the decision of our provincial supervisor." Chant's sincere belief was that Hôtel-Dieu would continue to provide excellent care and compassion to its patients. He praised the staff for "the fine and professional" work, and added, "I am thankful for my successful career in serving the health care sector for 34 years, the last 18 of which as CEO. I remain proud of the people I have worked with and all that we have accomplished." Deane, too, applauded the "top quality care" that Chant provided the hospital.

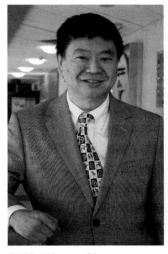

2009, Warren Chant

Dr. Percy Demers

In September 2011, Hôtel-Dieu Grace Hospital paid tribute to the late Dr. Percy Demers by naming its cardiac centre after him. During the dedication ceremony, hospital staff, family, friends and colleagues gathered to mark the event where a plaque was mounted on the 4th floor.

The newly named Dr. Percy Demers Cardiac Centre, to be located in the new Ambulatory Care and Outpatients Services Centre, will include: The Anthony F. Fuerth Cardiac Care Unit; 4 Medical/Telemetry Ward; Cardiac Catheterization/Angioplasty; Cardiac Diagnostics and the Arrhythmia/Pacemaker Clinic.

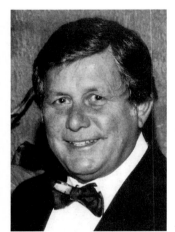

Dr. Percy Demers

The amiable Dr. Demers is regarded as a legendary figure in the history of the hospital. His roots with Hôtel-Dieu ran deep. He started at the hospital in 1960, and continued until 2002. For eight of those years this cardiac specialist was the chief of medicine.

"Dr. Demers was an extraordinarily gifted and compassionate healer who devotedly attended to the needs of his patients and their families," said Ken Deane, the hospital's CEO. He went on to say that Dr. Demers was "a valued mentor and friend to cardiac caregivers and staff. He will forever be remembered for his leadership in establishing a cardiac care program of excellence for the residents of Windsor-Essex."

The year following the special dedication, another tribute to Dr. Demers took place. In 2012, in recognition of "Doctor's Day," a day set aside to honour doctors in places all over the world, Hôtel-Dieu Grace announced a new annual award to recognize excellence in care by physicians. The first of these went to Dr. Jack Speirs, an interventional radiologist and Interim Chief and Medical Director of Hôtel-Dieu Grace Hospital's Diagnostic Imaging Department, has been selected as the inaugural recipient of.

The award, "The Dr. Percy Demers Physician Excellence Award" was aptly named in honour of Dr. Demers, because it honors physicians who demonstrate the kind of commitment and dedication to excellence in medical care that he had shown in his own career.

A panel of five Hôtel-Dieu Grace physicians from various medical disciplines selected Dr. Speirs from a hundred nominations. "All the nominees are deserving of the award, however, Jack was the clear choice," commented Dr. Gord Vail, HDGH Chief of Staff. He said Dr. Speirs was "an amazing specialist whose great skills have benefited many patients in our community. In working with the medical staff and caring for patients, he is dedicated, selfless and a real inspiration."

Dr. Speirs has worked at HDGH since 1998 and practices a sub-specialty that is often referred to as miracle medicine. Using HDGH's advanced diagnostic imaging equipment, he is able to perform minimally invasive procedures to remove blockages to arteries and coiling of brain aneurisms.

Speirs he said that when he started at Hôtel-Dieu in 1998, Dr. Demers was "already a legend."

He added, "To be named by my peers for an award in his honour is very humbling and a tremendous privilege."

In June of 2013, Dr. Frank DeMarco, past president of the Essex County Medical Society, and a former clinical trial investigator, was given the award. He worked at Hôtel-Dieu from 1960 to 2002, specializing in the care of acutely ill hospitalized patients. He continues to run a family practice on Walker Road, and is an adjunct professor at the Schulich School of Medicine's Windsor campus.

"Dr. DeMarco is passing on his extensive knowledge of medicine to our future doctors. It is a privilege to honour Frank's dedication to his field with this award," said Dr. Vail said, who was responsible for coming up with the idea for this award.

When he first proposed this way of honoring doctors, he maintained that it was traditional for hospitals to offer awards of excellence in nursing and to long-term service workers but there was nothing specifically for physicians at Hôtel Dieu.

"This annual award will be an opportunity to highlight a top physician at Hôtel Dieu," said Vail, "It may be a physician known to the community, or little known. It could recognize

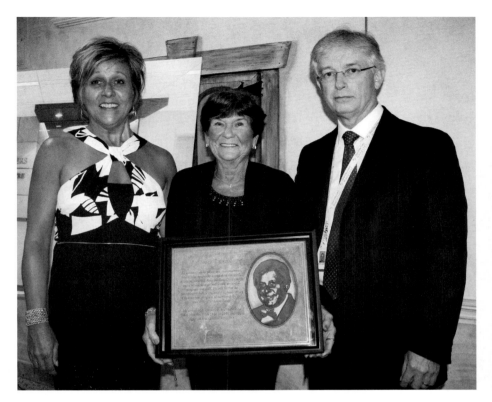

2011, Percey Demers dedication

many years of service; a unique skill set; above-and-beyond approaches to patient care; or a combination of these and other factors."

A bursary of $2,000 in Dr. Demers' name is also awarded annually to a medical student who best exemplifies the attributes of collegiality, teamwork, trustworthiness and patient focus.

Hotel-Dieu Grace Foundation

Bill Marra is president of the Hôtel-Dieu Grace Foundation, an organization started in 2005, and created to help fund the hospital's ability to pay for capital and equipment needs.

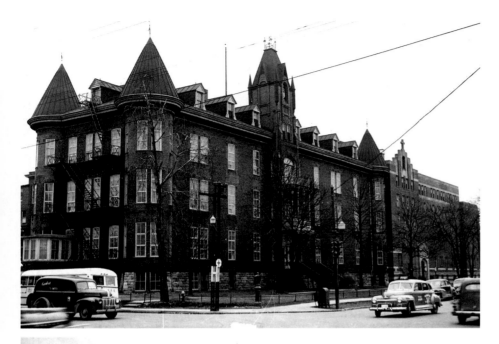

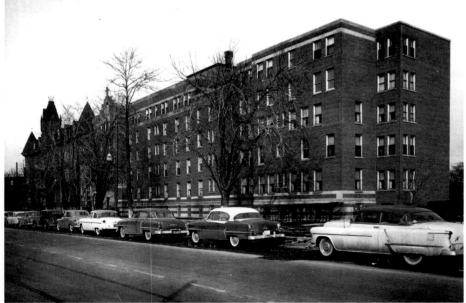

Hôtel-Dieu: top, 1890; bottom, 1938

This veteran city councillor probably knows his way around the hospital better than most, having started working there in 1982 when he was still in high school. He was hired as a dishwasher, but also served food to the patients, washed the carts, and scrubbed pots and pans by hand. Eventually he moved into the kitchen where he started cooking.

"They found out I was a short order cook at Franco's (restaurant), and so they trained me to work as a cook here as well," said Marra, now a city councillor. "I was able to train under some very talented cooks and chefs. I didn't realize how valuable that experience was until later in life." Marra regarded them as mentors. Among them was Sister Laporte. He recalled her as "a very disciplined person" but also someone who had a keen interest in how her employees were doing.

"She wanted to know if I was getting my work done, and asked about my family. I truly came to love Sister Laporte. She was strict and demanding, but she cared about us, and we needed that kind of guidance."

But there were moments when there was some tomfoolery. "Like the food fights in the kitchen. One morning someone came in and discovered a bunch of eggshells where eggshells shouldn't be. There were a few times I thought I would lose my job, but sister was good enough. She was very unhappy and let us know, but she knew we were young and we exercised poor judgment and she just reminded us how fortunate we were to have the jobs we did."

Marra left the hospital in 1988 when he embarked on his career in the Criminal Justice field. From 1997 to 2011, he served as the Executive Director of New Beginnings, which provides residential and non-residential Children and Youth Services in Windsor and Essex County. Marra's earlier involvement with the hospital eventually led him back to Hôtel-Dieu where he was appointed to its board of directors. "I thought it was a wonderful privilege, and I wanted to stay involved in my community…The experience rekindled my "love affair with the institution that I had grown up in as a teenager."

Marra also served as chair of the Hôtel-Dieu Grace Hospital Board, and was a founding member of that Hospital's Foundation. In September 2011, Councillor Marra was asked to be President and Executive Director of the Hôtel-Dieu Grace Hospital Foundation. Through his efforts with this organization, he has managed to dispense some $4.4 million to buy medical equipment and supplies. Since 2006, the Foundation has raised over $15 million.

The Last Ones

They landed in Windsor at the end of a humid summer in 1888. Slightly more than 120 years later, the descendants of this historic religious order started to pack up to depart the city, and leave behind a legacy of work among the sick.

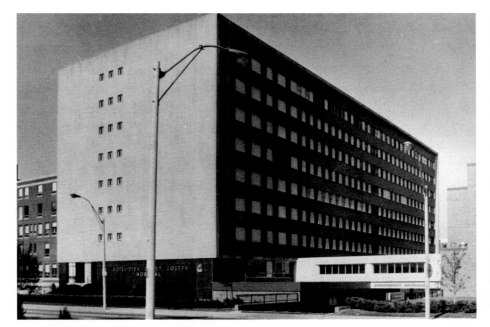

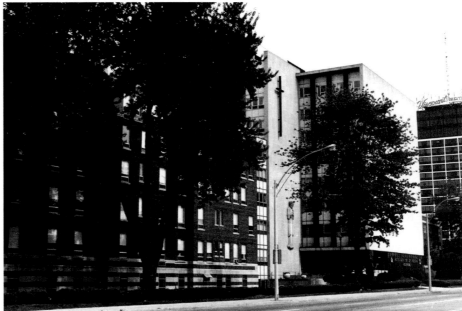

Hôtel-Dieu: top, 1962; bottom, 1982

185

Religious Hospitallers of St. Joseph 2009, left to right: Sr. Marguerite Laporte, Sr. Rose-Marie Dufault, Sr. Bernice Bondy, Sr. Angelina Duguay, Sr. Cecile LeBoeuf, Sr. Aurore Beaulieu

There were five sisters from Montreal who disembarked the train down by the river in Windsor in 1888, and began their work of building a hospital here.

In the spring of 2009, there were six heading out to join others in their religious communities now residing in convents in Montreal and Kingston. They left behind a lifetime of memories. The six were now elderly and retired, and the hospital their founders had started had changed dramatically. It was no longer the same place, this Hôtel-Dieu that towers over Ouellette Avenue. One hundred and twenty years before them at the corner of Erie and Ouellette, its foundress, Mother Pâquet, nurtured the vision of building a facility that would serve this community for years to come. Indeed, it did, and it continues that work.

But the Religious Hospitallers of St. Joseph's General Council thought it best to withdraw the sisters who still resided in the city. It didn't see replacing them. The order's Superior General Sister Marie-Therese Laliberte informed Hôtel-Dieu interim CEO John Coughlin that sisters Cecile LeBoeuf, Aurore Beaulieu, Marguerite Laporte, Bernice Bondy, Angelina Duguay and Rose-Marie Dufault would be the last ones to serve there.

"We very much regret having to leave Windsor where the congregation has laboured since 1888," Laliberte told *The Windsor Star*. At that point in time, the religious sisters were no longer assigned to any official roles in the hospital's day-to-day operations, but, like their predecessors, they worked tirelessly as volunteers. Coughlin also said they provided "a comforting presence to many patients." He told *The Star*, "It's very sad for us to see the sisters leave. Some of the sisters have spent quite a bit of time with our renal patients...they also attend mass, which is televised to the patients. The elderly patients who grew up in Windsor with Hôtel-Dieu and are used to the way it was in the old days...They do appreciate the visits from the sisters and will miss that."

Like other religious orders, the Religious Hospitallers have struggled to maintain a healthy membership. No candidates are stepping forward. Sisters LeBoeuf (the last sister to serve as CEO) and Beaulieu both said upon their departure how they would miss the community they've served for more than 60 years.

And when they left in 2009, ironically these six sisters were still owners of the hospital, and continued to wield corporate reserve powers, such as deciding upon the choice of the hospital's CEO and board appointments. But this arrangement was changed when the sisters transferred that authority to Catholic Health International, a public body incorporated under both civil and canon law. Each congregation—like the Religious Hospitallers of St. Joseph—is represented on the board of Catholic Health International.

The Six Who Made That Final Exit

Sister Rose-Marie Dufault

Sister Rose-Marie Dufault arrived at Hôtel-Dieu in 1965. She worked with the emergency physicians to develop a Code Blue team. She was responsible for introducing and creating the first Cardiac Care Unit at the hospital. Besides being Director of Nursing, Sister Dufault served on the Hôtel-Dieu Board of Directors. Other positions she held were Vice President of Mission Services and Pastoral Services and the Liaison to the Healthcare System for the Religious Hospitallers of St. Joseph. Sister Dufault has also been the chronicler of the Hôtel-Dieu sisters, and has continued to be in charge of preserving the artifacts for the order.

Sister Marguerite Laporte

Sister Laporte was from St. Joachim. She was 21 when she entered the convent at Villa Maria, but she spent her first five years in Whitelaw, Alberta where the religious order operated a hospice for elderly patients. For the next four years, Sister Laporte worked at the Mother and Provincial Houses for the Religious Hospitallers of St. Joseph in Montreal. Along the way, she acquired knowledge in kitchen management, and was assigned to supervising and scheduling the meal preparations for patients, staff and board functions at Hôtel-Dieu. Sister Laporte spent 30 years working in this field.

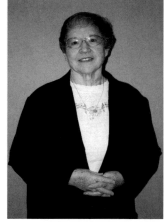

Sister Marguerite Laporte

Sister Angelina Duguay

Sister Angelina entered the order in Montreal. For the next 38 years, she worked out of that city's Hôtel-Dieu where she was Director of Linen and Laundry Services and Director of Volunteers. She was also the Assistant Superior at the Mother House for six years. When she retired, she relocated to Windsor at Villa Maria Home for the Aged. For two years, she assisted with the fundraising before moving to the Hôtel-Dieu Grace convent. There she served as Superior for three years. Sister Duguay was instrumental in making the arrangements for the move to Kingston and closing the community in Windsor.

Sister Aurore Beaulieu

Sister Aurore entered the religious order in 1942, and worked entirely in Windsor at Hôtel-Dieu following her graduation from its School of Nursing. Her job was in the Radiology Department where eventually she became a certified X-ray technician. Sister Beaulieu went on to be director of the X-ray department for 20 years. In 1974, Sister Beaulieu developed a different approach for helping patients make that difficult transition from the hospital to care in the community. After her retirement, Sister Beaulieu volunteered, visiting patients in the Renal Dialysis Unit at Hôtel-Dieu.

Sister Bernice Bondy

Sister Bernice Bondy hailed from Anderdon Township near Amherstburg. She entered the convent at Villa Maria in Windsor when she was 20. She worked as the hospital convent's housekeeper. Eventually, she trained to become a nurse's aide, and for the first 10 years in that position, she served in the Med-Surg Unit, then later with the chronically ill patients in Chronic Care. From 1994 to 2000 Sister Bondy was Superior of the nuns at Hôtel-Dieu.

Before departing the hospital and Windsor, she worked briefly at Villa Maria.

Sister Cecile LeBoeuf

Sister LeBoeuf was 25 when she entered the convent, and served as the CEO of the hospital from 1965 to 1968. She worked in Cardiac Investigations with Dr. Percy Demers for 18 years where she assisted with the administration of outpatient stress tests. After leaving her job of running Hôtel-Dieu she volunteered for 12 years at Villa Maria.

The Province Steps In

Ken Deane was appointed by the McGuinty Government as Hôtel-Dieu Grace Supervisor in January 2011, and immediately assumed full powers of the hospital board. His role was to work closely with senior officials and the Erie Health Integration Network to ensure that hospital management and staff were working together effectively in the best interest of patients.

In 2011 at the Ontario Hospital Association Health Achieve Conference, the soft-spoken and mannered Deane delivered a presentation to a group that was a slice of the media coverage surrounding his hospital. Much of it reached back to coverage of the Lori Dupont tragedy as well as the surgical errors and investigations. Deane wasn't out to expose anyone, or remind anyone. His motive was simple:

"I wanted the audience to have an appreciation for being a staff member here and being in the community, and reading about this and having an appreciation for the profound impact it could have on staff and on the public. The cumulative impact had to be profound on a subconscious level. And for staff? They were in the media all the time…I think what has been lost in people is appreciation for and understanding of this organization."

Deane's ability to present, of course, was honed from many years of being involved in professional and educational activities, primarily from presenting at numerous conferences and writing several management articles and serving on boards and committees in social services and health care. Deane also brought a wealth of experience from working with numerous health reorganization teams. As one Hôtel-Dieu spokesperson said, "He knows how to talk to people—he can relate to them, knows how to listen."

It may be this approach that defines the way Ken Deane runs an organization. It also echoes those early years of Hôtel-Dieu when the nuns learned to keep their ear to the ground, and find the ways to calm their worries. Deane, however, is one to confront the challenges honestly and directly. The same could be said for many of the Superiors who led this hospital through the 1920s and 1930s. That has also meant putting faith in individuals, recognizing human frailty, forgiving mistakes, but mostly moving on, moving ahead, and embracing values.

Deane's grasp of the past and the future of Hôtel-Dieu Grace is better than most. He was its Chief Executive Officer from 2002 to 2004. He also brought with him the vast experience of working as the Shared Chief Operating Officer of London Health Sciences Centre and St. Joseph's Health Care in London. He was also seconded to the province in 2008 to work as Assistant Deputy Minister in the Ministry of Health. This return to Windsor now meant reporting directly to the Minister of Health, who wanted to use his experience in the health field to address relationship and cultural issues and to oversee implementation of the recommendations for Hôtel-Dieu Grace that had been stipulated in the provincial report on the controversial surgical and pathology issues at local hospitals.

"I have full confidence in Mr. Deane," said Deb Matthews, then Minister of Health.

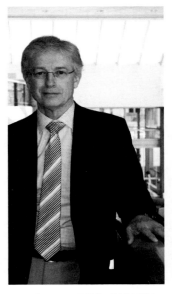

Ken Deane, CEO of HDGH

"He will ensure that the recommendations from the *Report of the Investigators of Surgical and Pathology Issues at Three Essex County Hospitals* are implemented as quickly as possible, with the best interest of patients in mind. I want people in Windsor to know that they can count on receiving high quality care at the Hôtel-Dieu Grace Hospital."

Deane embraced the challenges and told *The Windsor Star:* "I'm looking forward to the challenge of working with everyone at the Hôtel-Dieu Grace Hospital. I will be very clear about what we're going to accomplish and then empowering people to do their jobs."

His popularity was evident at Hôtel-Dieu Grace; it prompted a petition from the staff urging the Ministry of Health to allow Deane to stay on as CEO once the provincial supervision period ended. And that occurred. Carol Derbyshire, chair of the Hôtel-Dieu Grace advisory board said, "In order to capitalize on the momentum and significant gains made over the past 18 months, the Board agreed that an offer would be made to Ken." Now Deane moves to the next chapter in the saga of Hôtel-Dieu Grace, once again finding a way to ensure its future.

The Final Chapter

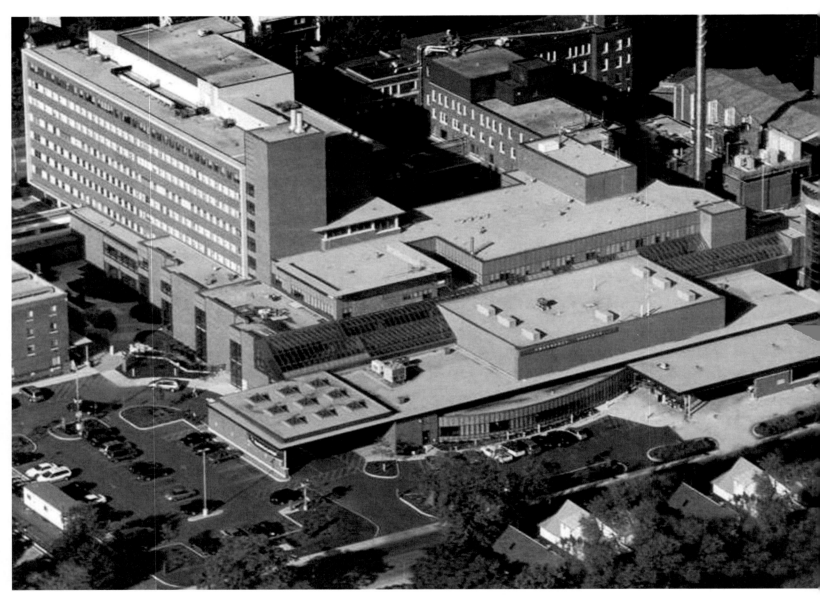

An Aerial shot of Hôtel-Dieu Grace Hospital: Ouellette tower at left, Emergency entrance lower right

Transforming Health Care
in our Community

Luann Kapasi, Senior Communications Officer
Hôtel-Dieu Grace Hospital

WHEN SISTER AURORE BEAULIEU APPROACHED ME IN JANUARY 2012 WITH A REQUEST TO HAVE A book written to mark the hospital's 125th anniversary, I had no idea that the final chapter would look like this. At that time, I expected the hospital to go on for the next 125 years caring for acute care patients much the same as it had done in the past. But, an announcement in April 2012 by the Provincial Government suggesting that Windsor's two existing facilities be replaced with a state of the art, single site acute care facility, has moved us in a completely new direction. We are now looking at a future that will transform health care for the benefit of our community, one in which Hôtel-Dieu Grace will play a very different role, but an important one.

The Windsor Hospitals Study Task Force, which included former MPP and Cabinet Minister Dave Cooke, former city councilor Tom Porter and MPP Teresa Piruzza, officially launched their public consultation process in July 2012 with a plan to submit a final report to the province by November, 2012 which would include a recommendation whether to move forward into the next phase. The task force met with staff at all three hospitals in Windsor-Essex, their Boards, long–term care homes, the university and college, the LHIN, labour representatives and community service providers.

According to the Windsor Hospitals Study, three main questions were at the centre of public conversation regarding a new facility:

- Would there be an improvement to the delivery of acute care services in the region with a new, single site acute care hospital?

- Would a new facility be a good value for the money?

- What other considerations must be addressed if the community is in support of the new hospital?

After five months of public consultations, the Windsor Hospitals Study Task Force presented their final 16 page report on December 7, 2012. The report which was sent to the provincial ministers of health and finance indicated that there was strong community interest in a single site acute care hospital and recommended that the provincial government should proceed immediately in approving the planning and construction of a new single-site acute care hospital. The task force said that they heard clearly from the community that a new single-site state-of-the-art acute care facility is needed, wanted and the best step forward for the community.

According to the task force, the province would have to spend about $1.8 billion on new capital projects just to keep the two existing hospitals going for the foreseeable future, and a brand new state-of-the-art facility would cost between $800 million and $1.5 billion. For many it appeared that the decision was clear. A state of the art single site acute care hospital is what this community needs and deserves.

Once that decision was made, the government immediately provided $2.5 million in funding to move forward with the capital planning process. The government also challenged our two local hospitals to resolve the governance of the new acute care facility before the capital planning process could begin. With that, the Board of Directors of both Hôtel-Dieu Grace Hospital and Windsor Regional Hospital recognized the challenge before them and created a clear focus on what would be in the best interest of the community and how best to move forward with the capital planning for a new state-of-the-art acute care hospital without delay.

On February 7, 2013, both hospital Boards agreed on a proposed new vision for health care delivery in Windsor that marked a significant and historic step on the road to a new state-of-the-art acute care hospital. In the interim, before the new acute care site is operational, services are being realigned making Windsor Regional Hospital responsible for all services at Metropolitan and Ouellette Avenue campuses. At the same time, Hôtel-Dieu Grace Hospital is responsible for all non-acute care services at, and related to the Tayfour Campus and retains oversight of the Community Crisis Centre.

The following are highlights of the resolution signed by the Boards of WRH and HDGH:

- WRH would be responsible for all acute care services – such as emergency treatment, acute inpatient services, intensive and critical care units, cancer care and outpatient services as required to support acute care services—at a new hospital site.

- HDGH would be responsible for all non-acute care services. This includes the Tayfour Campus site currently operated by WRH, with services such as chronic care, regional rehabilitation, specialized mental health and addictions, and children's mental health. Once the single site acute care hospital is operational, the existing Hôtel-Dieu Grace Hospital site on Ouellette could, if approved by the Erie St. Clair Local Health Integration Network and the Ministry of Health and Long term Care, be reconfigured to focus on non-acute services such as ambulatory care, urgent care, diagnostic services and day surgery.

The date established for the realignment of programs and services under the interim operating model for both hospitals has been set for October 1, 2013.

Moving to this Interim Operating Model on October 1, 2013, before moving to a new single-site acute care facility will make it possible to:

- Optimize capacity across both sites
- Re-balance activity across both sites
- Explore operating efficiencies with a higher critical mass of activity
- Explore opportunities for improved operating efficiency through economies of scale in administrative and support services
- Improve coordination and consistency in service delivery
- Facilitate best practices and models of care and standardization of both clinical and non-clinical processes and practices that have been shown to optimize the efficiency of acute care services
- Adopt a consistent city-wide approach to patient quality and safety
- Qualify for increased cancer funding
- Establish a single professional (medical/ dental/midwives) staff structure per hospital corporation
- A single unified professional staff, unified medical departments and a single Medical Advisory Committee (MAC) that will facilitate improved inter-site access to clinical consultation and clinical technologies
- Allow for Administration and professional staff to make day-to-day operational decisions and Boards to govern with a vision to the future
- Commence the detailed planning required before the eventual move to a new single acute care site

This is an exciting time for our community as healthcare history is being made once again through a vision agreed upon between the Board of Directors of Hôtel-Dieu Grace Hospital and Windsor Regional Hospital. According to an article by Beatrice Fantoni that appeared in The Windsor Star, April 21, 2012, a new state-of-the-art acute care facility is expected to have at least 700 beds (with room for expansion), 80 percent private rooms and 20 percent wards, 25 operating rooms and the capacity for 120,000 ER visits annually.

In effect, this realignment returns the organization to its roots, and its long-time vision and Mission: to heal, comfort and care for some of our most vulnerable citizens, including our elderly, those requiring rehabilitation, those who need long-term treatment for mental health issues, and those who need help recovering from addictions.

We have come a long way since the Sisters arrived here from Montreal in September, 1888 to look after the sick, the poor and with a secondary objective of teaching black children. They made history in Windsor when they arrived and purchased six vacant lots on Ouellette Avenue as the chosen site for Windsor's first hospital. They were here less than a month when construction began on October 14, 1888, to build a three-story hospital with a capacity of 100 beds. That was 125 years ago. As the Sisters saw the health care needs of the community change over the years, they endeavored to meet those needs—much the same as the Boards of Hôtel-Dieu Grace and Windsor Regional Hospital are doing today.